The Examined Illness

Global Health Humanities

Series Editors: Susan Hogan and Anna Greenwood
Print ISSN: 2752-8545 | **Online ISSN:** 2752-8553

Global Health Humanities series examines the health humanities from a number of perspectives, incorporating: medical humanities; health humanities; history of medicine; and arts and health. Contributions to the series focus on a wide range of subjects and utilise numerous methodologies and perspectives.

The series has multiple formats: traditional scholarly monographs; edited collections; and shorter format volumes. Authors include established scholars in the field, emerging early-career scholars, and practitioners. The series will appeal to health humanities scholars; clinicians and carers; and arts and humanities practitioners, as well as the learned general public.

In this series:

Making Sense of Medicine: Material Culture and the Reproduction of Medical Knowledge, edited by John Nott and Anna Harris (2022)
Fighting for the Soul of General Practice: The Algorithm Will See You Now, by Rupal Shah and Jens Foell (2023)
Drawing, Well-being and the Exploration of Everyday Place: 228 Sketches of Clifton Street, by Nicole Porter (2024)
The Examined Illness by Darrel Moellendorf (2026)

Faced with a life-threatening illness, philosopher Darrel Moellendorf explores the question important to all of us: How can we live well? *Writing with a rare blend of unflinching realism, humor, and tenderness, Moellendorf draws inspiration from philosophers, theologians, and poets (as well as Bruce Springsteen and Wile E. Coyote), offering an extraordinary meditation on our finitude, mortality, vulnerability, and need for true connections with others. This book ventures into deep terrain: What is hope and why is it important? How can we learn patience and courage? We witness that moments of deep delight are possible even under dire circumstances. This is a book filled with wisdom, yet earthy and engaging - never pedantic. A stirring and uplifting celebration of life. I didn't want to put it down.*

Alisa Carse, associate professor of philosophy and faculty affiliate of the Kennedy Institute of Ethics, Georgetown University

The Examined Illness: A Philosopher's Confrontation with Deadly Disease *is an important book. Philosopher Darrel Mollendorf offers us a moving and intimate account of his experience with illness. Anyone who has gone through this kind of trial or, like me, has accompanied a loved one through all the stages of the shattering diagnosis, the painful treatment, the miraculous remission, the dreaded relapse, the ultimate resort of transplantation, the undetermined convalescence, will be deeply stirred by this book. A philosophical reflection that will transport all readers into the concrete experience of mortality, grief, and even the social determinants of survival. Mostly, a memoir that speaks to us of love, hope, and the invaluable friendship of an aging dog.*

Ryoa Chung, professor of philosophy and co-director of the Centre de Recherche en Éthique/Center for Research in Ethics (CRE), Université de Montréal

Moellendorf is a man who has learned to live well in the face of death, and it's our good fortune that he recounts his journey, offering philosophical reflections.

Aaron James, professor of philosophy, University of California Irvine

An Examined Illness *is a window into what it is to experience serious, possibly terminal, illness. While this is a near universal experience - most of us will experience some form of serious illness ourselves, and if not, we will suffer with friends and family who do. Yet, in our society illness and death are largely hidden, not talked about, avoided at all costs. As a result, what illness is like is uncharted and diagnosis brings fear of the unknown. Moellendoft's account while unique to him, speaks directly to us all. He allows us to hear the patient's voice - to have a sense of what it is like to be ill - from the mundane impacts of tiredness and loss of taste, to the existential fear of losing ourselves. It is an amazing and necessary read.*

Heather Widdows, professor of philosophy, Warwick University

The Examined Illness *is a captivating, deeply moving work, beautifully told with sardonic wisdom and humour. Darrel Moellendorf is one of today's leading political philosophers and a talented writer. In 2016 he was diagnosed with the deadly blood cancer* myelofibrosis. *This book is the chronicle of the stem cell transplants that saved his life. The main part of the book was written and published first as a blog, in real time, expressing his hopes and fears, through diagnosis, preparation, treatment, recovery, then relapse, and repeat. Throughout, it is suffused with philosophical reflections, further developed in the Epilogue. It has already brought comfort and insight to many. Moellendorf's bravery in writing such a brilliant and open volume is an inspiration to us all. It is an intricate meditation on the theory and practice of hope.*

Jonnathan Wolff, emeritus professor of philosophy and public policy, Blavatnik School of Government, Oxford University

The Examined Illness

A Philosopher's Confrontation with Deadly Disease

Darrel Moellendorf

intellect

Bristol, UK / Chicago, USA

First published in the UK in 2026 by
Intellect, The Mill, Parnall Road, Fishponds, Bristol, BS16 3JG, UK

First published in the USA in 2026 by
Intellect, The University of Chicago Press, 1427 E. 60th Street, Chicago, IL 60637, USA

EU GPSR Authorised Representative
LOGOS EUROPE, 9 rue Nicolas Poussin, 17000, LA ROCHELLE, France
E-mail: Contact@logoseurope.eu

A catalogue record for this book is available from the British Library.

Copy editor and typesetter: MPS Limited
Cover designers: Natalie Thomas and Tanya Montefusco
Production editor: Tian Greaves

Hardback ISBN: 978-1-83595-324-2
Paperback ISBN: 978-1-83595-373-0
ePDF ISBN: 978-1-83595-326-6
ePUB ISBN: 978-1-83595-325-9

This is a peer-reviewed publication.

to Frank
without whom not

[L]anguage ... gives man the power to abstract from the concretely given and, after having abstracted from it, to return to it, to interpret and transform it. The most vital being is the being which has the word and is by the word liberated from bondage to the given.

-Paul Tillich, *The Courage to Be*

Contents

Acknowledgements

My deepest thanks go to Frank Keßler, to whom this book is dedicated, for saving my life. I am also immensely thankful to the transplant team at Goethe University Clinic for seeing me through the transplant: Professor Dr med. Hubert Serve, PD Dr med. Gesine Bug, Dr med. Fabian Lang, Argiri Tseviki, as well as the nursing, orderly, and custodial staff on the eleventh floor transplant unit. Their expertise and care are fabulous. I am also grateful to many friends and family members who offered support during the transplant and recovery, among them are Astrid, Bonnie, Chea, Daniel C., Daniel P., Dave, Don, Ellen, Emiel, Eszter, Gerrard, Ingrid, Jo-Al, Katrin, Kevin, Lara, Marino, Merton, Michael, Per, Rainer, Rebecca, Roger, and Teresa, among others. Farid and Brad kept my attention diverted from illness by involving me in interesting conversation throughout the period recorded here. The Unitarian Universalist Rhine-Main Fellowship helped clean our house so that I could return safely from the hospital. After I had recovered from the events described in this book and during my subsequent second illness and recovery, Andrea was a constant source of support and love. Although he will never read and understand the words, my life throughout this time has been deeply enriched by the companionship of Rex.

Finding a publisher for this book was not easy. It might never have been published if Tim Mitchell at Intellect Books and Anna Greenwood and Susan Hogan of the Global Health Humanities series at Intellect had not decided to take a chance on it. I am deeply grateful to them for believing in it. I am also grateful to the many people who read and offered feedback on parts of the manuscript over the past several years. These include Carlos Bermúdez, Gerrard Bester, Alisa Carse, Jeff Dean, Joanna Green, Bonnie Friedmann, Aaron James, Lisa Kessler, Don Kraemer, Hennie Lötter, Richard E. Miller, Kathy Robbins, Philipp Schink, and Jonathan Wolff. I presented parts of the text to nursing students at the University of Johannesburg. I would like to thank Hennie Lötter for organizing the event. I also discussed a few chapters of the book with students in Nicole Hassoun's course at Binghamton University. Many thanks to her for the opportunity. And I am grateful to the Philosophische Gesellschaft Basel for the opportunity to present a talk on themes from the book. I am deeply thankful to Ellen Nieß, who offers me invaluable support at work. She held the

Lehrstuhl together in my absence and helped me find the time to finish this project. Additionally, I am very grateful to Ella Gierß, who helped me tremendously with proofreading and preparing the text for publication. I am also grateful to Tian Greaves and Jessica Lovett for their helpful editorial assistance. And I am grateful to Marino Friedmann for the companionship and the astute advice regarding the subtitle.

Introductory Note

This book is a chronicle of, and reflection on, my first experience of a rare form of blood cancer called *myelofibrosis*. To save my life, I required and received a stem cell transplant. A transplant is as easy as receiving a blood transfusion. But prior to the transplant, the body must be prepared with several consecutive days of chemotherapy, which is directed at killing the existing bone marrow and immune system. That process leaves patients very weak and extremely vulnerable to infection. Once the transplant has been performed, the long process of regeneration begins. Initially, the biggest danger is the risk of deadly infection. Hence, patients are kept in extremely hygienic conditions where access is tightly controlled. Another danger is graft vs. host disease, which occurs when the new immune system attacks existing organs as foreign threats. This can be as benign as annoying rashes on parts of the body or as dangerous as threats to the functioning of the lungs. Recovery time from a stem cell transplant is usually between six and twelve months.

Most of this book was written in real time as I was diagnosed and treated for the cancer, and then also as I was in recovery. It was initially a blog written for family friends to keep them informed about my health status. The main part of the book is divided into three sections that correspond to the phases of diagnosis, treatment, and recovery. There is an epilogue that was written later; it offers some additional philosophical thinking about my experience with a very serious illness and life after that. The three sections written in real time have only been lightly edited after the fact for grammar, word choice, and accuracy. From the beginning of the project of converting the blog posts into a book, I have wanted to give voice to that experience as it was happening without substantial content editing later. This is based on my conviction that we have something to learn from persons experiencing illness, something that can be lost with too much reflective distance from the experience. This is not to say that reflection after the fact is unimportant. Some readers might find the epilogue to be the most interesting part of the book. But my view is that such reflection should not replace the voice of the patient as they are trying to come to terms with the illness. My hope is that other patients will find this book helpful, and that their friends and loved ones will as well. But illness is something that befalls us all, so the book is in fact for everyone.

Introductory Note

At the time of the transplant, I had been a professor of philosophy for 29 years. While that had been my profession, the origin of philosophy as an activity is with practitioners who thought of it as a way of life. Ever since Socrates, philosophy has been associated with the examined life. The earliest western philosophers were convinced that such a life was noble and the path to freedom and happiness. If indeed there are benefits of the examined life, these don't disappear when one becomes seriously ill. Quite the contrary, I think, and so this book is a chronicle of an examined illness.

Part I
Diagnosis

1
First Thoughts and Second Opinions

In late April 2016, I went to see my haematologist for a follow-up appointment. I had been seeing a haematologist regularly for the past eighteen years, ever since I had been diagnosed with a rare disease of the bone marrow called *essential thrombocythemia*. The primary manifestation of that disease is elevated blood platelets. In my case, that had been kept under control, and I had been otherwise asymptomatic, except for anaemia that had developed over the previous eight or so years.

I've lived in a few different countries, pursuing work as a professor of philosophy; and I've seen my share of haematologist/oncologist offices with waiting rooms often populated with visibly sick people, sometimes ashen and weak and occasionally wearing protective surgical masks. I never much enjoyed visiting the doctor, being confronted by the serious illness of others, and being reminded of my own disease. Although I taught philosophy, I did not have what might be called a philosophical attitude towards my own mortality. But after a hundred or so visits to these offices, I had become more or less accustomed to it.

This appointment was different. It followed up on one that I had a couple of weeks earlier during which my doctor, a squat man whom I often saw trotting from one examination room to the next, had administered a bone marrow biopsy on me in order to have a looksee at the state of the underlying disease. That biopsy had been the third in eighteen years.

It would be an understatement to call bone marrow biopsies unpleasant. A doctor uses a needle to pierce the tissue on the back side of the hip in order to gain access to the pelvic bone. The needle is twisted one way and then the other as it is pushed toward the bone. Although the tissue can be numbed, the bone cannot. Apparently, there is no way to get the biopsy needle into the bone and to the marrow other than simply driving very hard, again with the twisting motion, until the biopsy needle pierces the bone. To speak of it as a 'needle' might leave the wrong impression. It is hollow to allow for the collection of the marrow. But the stainless-steel shaft has to be strong enough to pierce bone, and robust enough not to buckle under the pressure applied to jam it into the bone. The needle has a handle at a right angle to the shaft made to be grabbed by the fingers and palm. The handle facilitates the required twisting motion. The original Jamshidi™ needle boasts a knob at the top, a protuberance of blue, industrial-strength polymer. Once the needle is forced in about an inch and a half, the inner core of the needle is removed and then the 360-degree twisting action begins. People sometimes talk of undergoing surgery as going under the knife. I like to think of having a bone marrow biopsy as going under the corkscrew.

Fortunately, there is little that can go wrong. So, other than anticipating the unanaesthetized bone pain, the immense discomfort of the pressure needed to drive the needle into the bone, and the weirdness of the twisting, I had very little to worry about on that day. As the doctor pushed and twisted the needle into the bone, he and the nurses chatted away about a football game the night before. 'Don't forget about the needle sticking out of my hip,' I wanted to say. But I refrained and braced myself for more pressure. Once the needle had been rammed to the marrow, its inner core was removed. More twisting. The marrow filled into the hollow cylinder. More soccer chat. As the needle was finally removed, part of my soul seemed to be sucked away. With the game fully analysed, they sat me up, ensured that I was steady on my feet, and dispatched me, only slightly dazed, homeward.

When my doctor ordered the bone marrow biopsy, I assumed that he was not driven purely by curiosity. I had been informed early in the treatment of *essential thrombocythemia* that one risk was that it might transform into *secondary myelofibrosis*, which involves bone marrow scarring that inhibits the production of blood cells. If you are accustomed to thinking of your longevity in terms of decades, with *myelofibrosis*, you have to reorient to thinking in terms of years. The process can be slowed a bit by medication, but the only cure is a stem cell transplant. Given that anaemia can be an indication for *myelofibrosis*, and that fibrosis can be seen from a marrow sample, I had a reasonably good hunch what my doctor was looking for.

That day in late April was sunny, the sort that lightens my spirits. The sun doesn't shine nearly often enough for me up here north of the 50th parallel north. Too many years spent in the subtropics have left me constitutionally ill-prepared for the days and days of cloudiness. I enjoyed the sunshine as I walked to my doctor's office for the follow-up appointment. Once there, I had my blood drawn as usual and waited to be called into his office. In his office, we did the routine survey of the results of the bloodwork. Nothing remarkable there. The platelet counts were under control and the other counts were out of whack in my usual ways. I was as anaemic as ever, no more and no less than in recent history. He was advising me on when we should meet again, when I reminded him of what he seemed to forget, but I could not. The bone marrow biopsy during my previous appointment. Duly prompted, he sought the results and informed me without surprise that the indication was *myelofibrosis.* Calmly, I asked him about the prognosis; he was non-committal. It seemed to depend on how quickly my counts fell, and all we could do was monitor that. In the end, the scarring of the marrow that is *myelofibrosis* inhibits all blood production. The question is how long that would take. He couldn't say, really. And he gave no indication that there should be a therapeutic change. Then he made his way rapidly down the hall, a flash of a white lab coat disappearing into another office. I made an appointment for my next regular visit and left. On my walk home, the April sunshine was hard to notice for the fog of my confusion. What had just happened?

An established principle of bioethics is that there should be no unnecessary invasive procedures. My doctor had conscientiously sought more information; acquiring it was certainly invasive. It required more than the usual amount of discomfort, but afterwards he did nothing with the information he gained. Something is wrong with this picture? Is the diagnosis not as bad as I had imagined? But then why do the biopsy, if positive results don't mandate some sort of change of care? When I got home, the internet offered confirmation that the diagnosis was just as bad as I had thought and although a stem cell transplant might offer the hope of a once-and-for-all cure, it was risky, and not an option for many patients. How long did I have? I couldn't even hazard a guess. More than a year, I reckoned, but perhaps not long enough to see my son graduate from high school or from college, and probably not long enough to reach retirement.

It did me no good to wonder without better answers than those that the doctor had given me. So, I decided to seek a second opinion. I emailed the head of Haematology at the medical school of my university. He answered promptly, reassured me, and was happy to conduct an examination and offer a second opinion. Thus, began my experience of being a stem cell transplant patient.

2 Healthcare for All Pt. 1

At the first meeting with the head of Haematology, I was pleased that he wanted to do more testing. And I was impressed that he ordered a change of medication. But it caused me to wonder all the more why the previous doctor had altered nothing after performing a bone marrow biopsy and changing my diagnosis. Did he think there was little point in doing anything else? Or, for some reason, did he really think 'wait and see' was the best approach? Did he just not know enough? But then why not he send me to someone else who knew more? Or did he not know enough to know that he didn't know enough?

For at least sixteen years, I had taken a medication called *Anagrelide*, which inhibits the production of blood platelets. I started *Anagrelide* shortly after its introduction to the market. When I had the opportunity to take it, I was eager to do so because the very first medication that I had taken, *hydroxyurea*, was not recommended for men trying to become fathers.

Anagrelide seemed not to cross into the semen. That meant that my wife and I could pursue our plan of having a child. By this time, I had been taking *Anagrelide* since before my son was born. At 16, he'd become taller than his mother, and nearly as tall as me. Innovations in medicine had made our family possible.

The new meds prescribed by my colleague are called *Jakavi* in Europe. The generic name is *ruxolitinib*. It had only been in the market for a few years. Here is what the European Medicines Agency says about it:

> *[R]uxolitinib* works by blocking a group of enzymes known as Janus kinases (JAKs), which are involved in the production and growth of blood cells. In *myelofibrosis* and *polycythaemia vera*, there is too much JAK activity, leading to the abnormal production of blood cells. These blood cells migrate to organs including the spleen, causing them to become enlarged. By blocking JAKs, *Jakavi* reduces the abnormal production of blood cells, thereby reducing the symptoms of the diseases.
>
> (European Medicines Agency n.d.: n.pag.)

I took my prescription for Jakavi to the pharmacist. He typed something into a computer and then informed me that he would have to place an order for it. He looked up at me quizzically. Did I realize how much my insurance was being charged for this? No. 'Over 4200 Euros', he said. And that was just for a 25-day dosage. Gulp. 'How much do I pay?' 'Ten Euros', he said, smiling.

3
Patients and Patience

After I made the appointment for the second opinion with the head of Haematology at my university, I had to wait. That, of course, gave me plenty of time to exercise my imagination. From what I had read on the internet, I knew that not everyone was a candidate for a stem cell transplant. If I was not a candidate, the disease would finally take me, but that would probably not be soon. Still, the end would not be pretty. 'Wasting away', it's called.

While waiting, I wrote a few letters to my son for safekeeping. Years ago, when my own mother died of a bone marrow disease, I was 23. I had not lived at home for several years. Still, I remember feeling like I never really got to know her as an adult. I had only known her through child and adolescent eyes. I still have a sense of loss about that. I expected my son would feel this all the more so if I were to die when he was merely a teenager. So, I decided to try writing letters to an adult version of him. One of the thoughts that I had at that time became a source of resolve. The disease might take away our future together, but we won't let it ruin our present. There is something perverse about letting worry about future loss render you unable to enjoy what you don't want to lose while you still have it.

Nonetheless, sometimes my imagination would outstrip what I understood to be the rational approach. I had begun, strangely, to experience the night sweats that I read about as possible symptoms; the fatigue from the anaemia became really noticeable for the first time. I attended a conference in southern California - a place I was very happy to visit, having lived many years there - and I was not much interested in socializing. I even found myself resting more often in the hotel room than strolling on the beach. I had begun to feel an enlarged spleen that I had read helps to produce blood in response to the scarring in the bone marrow that inhibits blood production there. I was sufficiently self-aware to consider that perhaps my imagination was getting the best of me. But I discarded that idea quickly as a failure to face up to reality. I was grimly resolved not to live in denial.

When I arrived for the consultation for the second opinion, my chest was tight. Sitting was uncomfortable due to the perceived enlarged spleen, and my blood pressure was through the roof. The head of Haematology led the consultation, and he was accompanied by a younger doctor, who worked in his unit. The head doctor was kind, affable, and calming. He assured me that there were options and, when I asked, he expressed confidence that I would see my son graduate from high school.

'The results of the previous bone marrow biopsy indicated an advanced stage of the disease, but they were inconclusive in some respects,' he said. I gritted my teeth when he recommended a second biopsy. He also recommended an ultrasound of the spleen to determine what I knew to be its enormous size. It was clear to me that the spleen was gorging. And what was up with my kidneys? Why was my creatinine level higher than normal? More testing was called for. More waiting.

One thought leads to another. But sometimes they do not lead out of the labyrinth of worry. Still, I had papers to grade, conferences to attend, writing deadlines to meet, my son's homework to supervise, our dog to walk, and family weekend outings to plan. John Lennon once sang 'life is what happens when you are busy making other plans'. It's also what happens when you are busy worrying about the future. Unfortunately, I was not always as rational as in the moment of clarity in writing the letters to my son: if one values life, it is irrational to be so consumed with anxiety about its end that one loses the joy of living. I am, of course, far from the first to have realized that.

In 23 BCE, the Latin poet Horace wrote a poem with the words Carpe Diem:

> In the moment of our talking, envious time has ebb'd away.
> Seize the present; trust tomorrow e'en as little as you may.
>
> (2004: Ode I:11)

About a half century later, Matthew 6: 34, reports Jesus saying, 'Take therefore no thought for the morrow: for the morrow shall take thought for the things of itself. Sufficient unto the day is the evil thereof' (1987). Another 100 or so years later, the Stoic philosopher Epictetus warned of the debilitating role of the imagination. 'Man is not worried by real problems so much as by his imagined anxieties about real problems' (Epictetus 1983: 5).

The ancient wisdom is sound advice for patients. Most of us are accustomed to living lives directed in significant measure by our own aims. We are agents. Sure, we have to follow the laws, do what the boss says, be polite, etc. But in liberal societies, adults have a great deal of scope to do as they want in the midst of these constraints. As patients, however, we may experience loss of control with regard to something that matters a lot to most of us, our health. We wait for test results. We let the doctors perform their curative attempts on us, and we wait and see what comes of it all. Typically, there is little that we can do to influence the result. In these cases, patience really is the best policy. Not that we can always exercise the kind of rational control over our fears that the counsel of patience recommends, but knowing that it is the rational policy that provides some leverage on our emotional responses.

Patient and *patience* have a common Latin root. Some people deny that we are ever so completely patients, without the capacity to influence outcomes significantly. They maintain that we can always affect the outcome, rather than simply wait for it to come or to be known.

Patience, they claim, is the counsel of defeatism. Instead, maintaining the right attitude towards the outcome helps to promote it. This is supposed to be the deep power of positive thinking.

There is a new age movie called *The Secret* that proclaims that maintaining a positive attitude causes health and riches.

But if you are a friend or family member of a patient, think carefully before you utter such a view to them. It's not just that the view is wishful thinking, although it is that. It's much worse. Consider the logic. If good fortune reliably comes to those with good attitudes, then those suffering ill fortune have at least in part brought it upon themselves. In some way or other, they must have failed to be sufficiently positive. The secret of *The Secret* is vicious victim blaming.

Having a good attitude is, without a doubt, crucially important. It's the carpe in carpe diem. The ancient counsel is to let go of our worries about the future because doing so lets us seize the day. The value of a good attitude is not its service in producing a better tomorrow. Rather, it's constitutive of enjoying the present.

The ultrasound showed that my spleen was only slightly enlarged, not all that much really, and importantly, not any more than it had been for the last several years. That's when a miracle of modern medicine occurred: Strangely, I stopped being able to feel my spleen! What I had been telling myself was grim resolve not to live in denial turned out to be the anxious workings of my own imagination.

I steeled myself for the second bone marrow biopsy. A doctor that I had not seen before, who seemed hardly old enough even to be in medical school, introduced herself. She escorted me into a room with a gleaming stainless-steel table and asked me to take off my shirt and pull down the waist of my pants to the point at which enough of my hip was exposed for her to get to work. She was all business. I lay there bracing myself. First, the cool spray of the topical disinfectant. Then the needle anaesthetizing the tissue. She was very short, so she had to lower the table to get the kind of leverage on the biopsy needle that she would need to pierce the bone. She drove the needle in. Grimace. She twisted it. And then it seemed as if she had decided to go on an exploratory mission. Was she heading off horizontally? More grimacing. The corners of my eyes were moist. She twisted the needle. She was working hard, and she was not satisfied. She was not finding what she was after. Finally, she asked, 'Did they get blood last time?' How the hell should I know, I wanted to say. But instead, I mustered a curt. 'I don't know'. Hmm. I wondered what it all meant. Could it be that my marrow was producing no blood at all? Finally, seemingly satisfied, she withdrew the needle and packed up. I pulled up my trousers and put on my shirt, and then I was invited to leave.

Up I stood, but too soon. The ground below me had transformed into a wave, and my legs were not surfing it well. As I headed to the waiting room, I resisted the strong temptation to sit down. I was not going to show any vulnerability, not there. I swerved to absorb the waves and headed down the hall. Where to? What next? I found a side corridor, and in it a vending machine. I leaned against it. Sugar ... chocolate would help. I fumbled for the money, bought the candy, stood leaning, and ate the candy. I weaved out of the hall, but a bit more steadily, down the corridor and out to the parking lot and my car, where I could sit alone for a few minutes.

Another week or two of waiting went by, during which I had time enough to entertain magical thoughts of spontaneous healing. But when I went in for the results, there was no magic. No miraculous recovery. Medical books would not be rewritten in light of the case of the philosopher whose disease inexplicably disappeared. The diagnosis from the previous bone marrow biopsy was confirmed. The *myelofibrosis* was in an advanced stage. I was in the upper section of the intermediate risk group. The median survival rate without a transplant was three years. The transplant had about a 70 percent success rate. The choice seemed clear. I could wait for a while for the transplant, but the longer I waited the more I would deteriorate, and the success rate of the transplant would fall correspondingly.

Was I even a candidate for a transplant? Was I healthy enough? What about my kidneys? What about that creatinine level? A transplant is tough on the kidneys. They have to process all the chemo that is sent to destroy the bone marrow. Then, if there is any trouble later with infections, the kidneys have to process the diagnostic fluid consumed to help identify where the infection is. I could perhaps end up dependent on dialysis. A nephrologist had to be consulted. I would need an ultrasound performed on my kidneys. I would have to wait and see if I were a candidate for transplant. And then even if I were a candidate, could a donor even be found?

In time, this all worked out.

I don't claim to have been a model Stoic during this final period of uncertainty, but I also wasn't a complete wreck. Life is what continued to happen. My wife and I went to a Bruce Springsteen concert. We had tickets for the standing section near the stage. The concert was like a huge tent revival, but for the faithful of many creeds and even of none. I stood with my Ray-Ban Wayfarers on. The guy next to me, at least two decades my junior, stood in his Misfits baseball cap and Aviator sunglasses. Ragtag communicants at the altar of rock 'n' roll, we sang along to every song. Often nearly shouting, but our voices didn't stand out. The entire audience was the choir. Then Springsteen hit the chorus of *No Surrender.*

> Once we made a promise, we swore we'd always remember no retreat, baby, no surrender.
>
> Blood brothers in a stormy night with a vow to defend. No retreat, baby, no surrender, no retreat, baby, no surrender.
>
> (Springsteen 1984)

Something warm was streaming under my sunglasses. I looked over at my brother in song, and I saw tears appear from under the bottom edge of his Aviators. Moved by the spirit, we sang as the band played on.

4 Father to Son and Back

I have dim memories of sitting in front of a TV with a rounded screen inside a blonde cabinet and rabbit ear antennae positioned on top. *Art Linkletter's House Party* is playing in black and white. The show regularly contained a segment in which children were interviewed. Invariably, they would say something cute and funny, which gave the segment its title, 'Kids Say the Darndest Things.' Later, Bill Cosby had a television show based on the same idea using the identical name. What made these shows especially entertaining was the unexpected nature of some of the responses. Sometimes a child would say something disarmingly honest that made Art or Bill stop in their tracks. Pause. And then the audience would explode into laughter.

When I was first diagnosed, the only person I told for several weeks was my wife. The ruse was up, however, when after attending several doctors' appointments during the work week, my administrative assistant found an appointment slip for a Haematologist. She didn't pry. But I knew that I was going to need her able help in juggling my schedule since the doctor's appointments were multiplying. Going to the doctor had become a part-time job. So, I told her. I then adopted the policy of telling people on a need-to-know basis. The first group consisted of close colleagues, siblings, and good friends. I was generally hesitant to tell people before I knew that a transplant was going to be available. How could I go back to them and say that there is no cure? I couldn't imagine it. So, whenever possible, I waited first to hear about the approval of the transplant and the identification of a donor.

I dreaded telling people about my diagnosis. In large part, this was because of the unpredictability of the responses. Sometimes I was thrust into the role of the therapist, having to set the grief-stricken person at ease. I was struggling enough with coming to terms with the diagnosis myself. Philosophical distance was not something I had attained. Occasionally, the message was easily and calmly absorbed. The person listened thoughtfully, expressed concern, asked good questions, and then we moved on. But in more than a few cases, it was much more difficult. Shock and anxiety would pour into the person's face. I could imagine them afterwards fumbling for their Xanax. My own precarious equilibrium could become unsettled by the conversation. Their shock was, of course, some cocktail of concern for me and their appreciation of their own vulnerability. The proportions would vary with each person.

I knew that I had to tell my son once it was relatively certain that I was a candidate for a stem cell transplant. The familiar dread returned. I steeled myself. My wife was away. After serving him one of his favourite dinners of fresh pasta and *panna cucina* sauce, I began, 'Remember how we sometimes talk about my anaemia.' Between forkfuls, I conveyed a few of the details of the treatment, induced immune system death via chemotherapy, hospitalization, surgical masks, long recovery, decent prospects of a cure, and the whole business. With his mouth full, he paused, reflected, and said, 'Oh, it's like AIDS caused by chemotherapy.' He swallowed and shovelled in another bite. I gulped. 'Uh, yeah ... I guess you could say that.' I hadn't really thought of it that way, and I was not particularly eager to do so. But, given my limited knowledge of the course that AIDS runs, I had to admit that it seemed about right.

I was anxious about the next move of the dialectic. He was processing. 'When is this going to happen?' 'Well, maybe not for another six months, maybe even a bit longer. We don't yet know exactly. I need a donor, and there's no big hurry.' He chewed and reflected again. 'Good, then I can procrastinate worrying.'

Done. The line was much longer than the ride. The conversation moved on to other topics.

I would have welcomed something stronger, but I was glad to have at least a glass of wine to drink as I reflected on his equanimity. I'd like to credit his parenting. But whatever the source, it had made things easy. And I was grateful. Procrastinate worrying. He made it sound so simple.

5
Give It up for Lent!

The Lenten period is when Christians are encouraged to reflect on their own limitations. In the midst of the hustle and bustle of life, the pain and inconvenience caused by giving up a pleasure or a minor indulgence brings the attention of the faithful back to their own finitude, embodiment, and mortality.

I don't think that I will have any trouble reflecting on my mortality this year; I'm giving up my immune system.

This coming Thursday - the day after Ash Wednesday - I check into the hospital, at which point I surrender myself to modern medical knowledge, the competence of my doctors and nurses, and the vagaries of complex biochemical processes. Surrender is just another part of being a patient.

Here's the plan. The treatment protocol assigns the days numerals that revolve around the transplant day. The days before the transplant have negative numerals, the days after have positive ones.

Give It up for Lent!

I arrive on day 7, and I am given an anticonvulsant. The chemo, it seems, can cause convulsions. I am also fitted with a port through which the chemo and stem cells will flow, the first to destroy and the second to rebuild. On days 6 through 3, I continue to receive the anticonvulsant supplemented by two different forms of chemotherapy, *busulfan* and *fludarabine*. These attack the immune system and immature blood cells. Three days of the regimen are sometimes used, but for the strong, a fourth day is preferred. The additional day better serves the purpose of killing the marrow, making the likelihood of a successful transplant greater.

According to the Wikipedia entry on *fludarabine*, 'Common side effects include nausea, diarrhoea, fever, rash, shortness of breath, numbness, vision changes, and feeling tired. Severe side effects include brain dysfunction, low blood cell counts, and lung inflammation' (2025: n.pag.). The doctors have assigned me a fourth day of chemo. I'm glad; I guess.

The point of the whole drill is to destroy my body's erstwhile best friend, my immune system. The mutinous forces of my bone marrow must be crushed and replaced with more benevolent ones.

Day 2 looks to be something of a respite. I receive only the anticonvulsant. On day 1, I received an immunosuppressant called *tacrolimus*, which targets T cells in my muscles. Produced by a soil bacterium, *tacrolimus* helps to reduce the incidence of organ rejection.

Meanwhile, my anonymous donor will be receiving daily injections of *filgrastim*, which causes the bone marrow to make and then release a whole bunch of stem cells into the blood. After several days of injections, the stem cells are harvested by a process called *apheresis*. Blood is removed and run through a machine; the stem cells are separated out, and the remaining blood is returned, all over the course of two to four hours. It could take a day or two to harvest enough stem cells from the donor. The result is the greatest gift that I could be given at this point in my life. I am filled with gratitude beyond measure for the generosity of that donor.

Day 0 is the transplant day. Almost anti-climatically, the stem cells are introduced into my body by means of an IV. By a mechanism of biochemical causation that I can't really fathom, the cells are propelled to my bones - I want to say that they seek my bones - where they squat in the residence that used to house my marrow. During days +1 to +6, I receive an additional immunosuppressant called *mycophenolate* to prevent rejection of the new bone marrow.

The first week or two after the transplant is critical. I will be in a condition known as *aplasia*. Absent any well-functioning bone marrow, my immune system will be in shambles. I will be dependent on blood transfusions. My job is simply to wait. The doctors look for signs that the stem cells are grafting and starting to make new bone marrow - this occurs 90 percent of the time. And I hope to avoid serious infection. My blood counts are continually monitored. When the new bone marrow produces enough blood for me to be safely released, I go home.

From start to finish, I can expect a five to six-week stay at the transplant unit. As I mentioned, I start on the day after Ash Wednesday, and I hope to be on my feet after Good Friday.

Part II
Inside

6

Day 7: The Countdown Begins

When the day began, it was still dark. I went downstairs to wake up my son for school. When I walked into the room, Rex, our family dog, greeted me like I had been gone for weeks. I was taken aback. He never does that in the morning. Uncanny. How did he know that I was leaving today? Rex will be all right. He has lots of humans who will take him for walks in the woods. He makes friends easily. He lives in the moment. As I write this, he's not wondering where I am. I think I will miss him much more than I will be missed. The inequality between species is not always to our advantage.

At the transplant unit, my wife and I were greeted by a remarkably friendly staff. A doctor and a nurse sat us down and explained various rules. I was given the first of several anticonvulsants, and I was put on a warning that the day would be full of information. But that's not all. They planned to perform a third bone marrow biopsy right away in order to get a baseline before the transplant. You could have heard my good cheer crash to the floor in whimpers. I tried to appear to take the news in stride, but I was not fooling anyone. The doctor said it was absolutely necessary. I was also to have a catheter inserted into me so that they could run all of the many fluids into me without re-poking me every time.

Then the nurse took us to my room. We entered an antechamber, where she inspected everything that I brought along: a laptop, a tablet, two ten-pound dumbbells, a yoga matt, several books, DVDs, eight pairs of sweatpants, eight long-sleeve v neck T-shirts - hospital chic - eight pairs of socks, and eight pairs of underwear - all previously washed per instructions at 60°C/140°F. Most of the DVDs were not allowed because the album that they were in would be too hard to disinfect. The same with an old book. Only new books are allowed. No yoga mats, because absolutely no time is to be spent on the floor. The computer, tablet, cell phone, cables, and weights were all swished with some kind of alcohol wipe.

I had an opportunity to peer into the room, my place of residence for the next five weeks. It is probably 12 feet by 15 feet, with a single bead, exercise cycle, TV, two monitors, a couple of stands that you might confuse for coat stands but are actually IV stands, and various devices that seem to read out measurements. All sorts of one-time use devices, wrapped in plastic and a couple of valves to which hoses apply. One seems to be for oxygen, not sure about the other one.

It was a bit harrowing to look in. It is most certainly a hospital room. And it is where I will live. My wife had to wear a gown and a face mask to enter. Once in the room, the nurse took my blood pressure and temperature - the latter I will have to do several times a day. I was weighed again my job twice a day. Then the nurse explained that they are vigilant against hospital bacteria. Every orifice except my ears - I mean *every one* - was to be swabbed and examined in the lab. Fortunately, there were two places that she left me to do in the privacy of the bathroom. I like her. She has a fine sense of humour about it all.

My instructions were then to shower, leaving the anti-bacterial soap on for at least two minutes before rinsing, and then put on my sweatpants and long-sleeved shirt. I was beginning to look the part of a patient. More rules: close the toilet top before flushing. Always wash hands with soap and then with disinfectant. If I drop something on the floor - where all the nasty germs live - I must call a nurse to pick it up. The floor is strictly verboten.

Then lunch came, but it deserves no further mention. As the doctor came in to perform the bone marrow biopsy and the catheter insertion, my wife conveniently used the opportunity to go buy some shower shoes for me, which we had forgotten. Bone marrow biopsies are almost routine affairs to me now. This doctor was competent. But I felt the deep, deep pain in the bone, nearly too much to take. She knew and backed off. She was also having trouble finding blood. She explained that it was due to the fibrosis, the scarring of the bone narrow. That might have gotten worse since May. The doctor got enough of what she wanted and withdrew the needle.

I was left to rest for a little while; then she came back with a tranquilizer, which I took before she inserted the catheter. By the time she started, I was a bit light-headed and certainly compliant. A hole in my neck was made first. Then 20 cm of tube were run into a vein almost as far as the heart. This way, the stuff they hook up to the catheter and drain into me will be taken directly to the heart and dispatched throughout my body right away. I have a master tube sticking out of my neck. It divides into four smaller tubes. As I write, I'm hooked up to two bags of saline solution. When I need to move around the room, I push the stand around like a dancing partner.

With the tube, the stand, and the bags, there is no denying now that I am a patient. The world of yesterday is gone. After all of these months of waiting, of worrying, of working at not worrying, it is really happening. I am a stem cell transplant patient. I have the tubes to prove it to myself and everyone else.

Day 7: The Countdown Begins

I texted a picture of me and my tubes to my sister. She replied, 'Just think of it as your cure starting.' I like that.

It's a long way from being over. One day at a time, I tell myself. Epictetus. Night has fallen. Tomorrow morning, I will awaken to a doctor who will start my chemotherapy regimen. It is really happening.

7

Day 6: Carpe Diem

From all I've heard, I'm on the downhill slide now, in terms of how I will feel and the risk level assumed.

Last night, I didn't sleep especially well. I had some discomfort from the tube and the biopsy site. But mostly I think it was simply the unfamiliar room. That it was a hospital room probably made it worse, but even when I travel for work and sleep in much nicer hotels, I usually have disrupted sleep.

Shortly after 6 a.m., having given up the battle with sleep, I hopped on the exercise cycle and rode it for 30 minutes while listening to Mudhoney's self-titled album. Nothing like a little high-octane grunge to get the body moving. As I was moving over to the dumbbells, the nurse came in with the first of my two daily bags of chemo. He had to start early because there must be three hours between the administration of each kind of chemo. They don't mix well apparently. I wasn't in the mood for a chemistry experiment, so we got started. Receiving my first-ever chemo treatment was pretty non-eventful, just like being hooked up to any ordinary bag of liquid.

The nurse then weighed me and took my temperature and blood pressure. The latter was high at 180, but that was due partially to riding. I saw no reason to let a little chemotherapy interrupt my workout. So, I spent about twenty minutes pushing and pulling the dumbbells.

Breakfast came. But the food was hardly worthy even of description.

After breakfast, I began to feel a bit dizzy. The nurse took my blood pressure again, but nothing was found that could have caused the dizziness. It was down to 160. Still too high. Later, he came in with the results of yesterday's blood test. The sodium and creatinine levels were also high. This has been a recurring theme throughout my treatment. It all points to the kidneys. But a couple of ultrasounds revealed nothing. And the creatinine, at least, has been high but stable for nearly ten years. Kidneys, however, are important for processing removal of chemo from the body. In my circumstances, any dysfunction of them is a concern. If they don't function well enough, dialysis might be needed.

The nurses hooked me up to a couple of bags of water over the course of the day, the better to flush the system with. And I have been drinking liquids almost continually, and ... well needing to visit the toilet every fifteen minutes or so. I have a name now for the fluid stand: Ginger Rogers. I push her around the room with her fluid bags when I need to visit the bathroom. On one occasion, I forgot to close the toilet lid before flushing. I broke the rules! I was paralyzed. No alarms went off! So, I took a deep breath, stepped back, and went about washing and disinfecting my hands.

My link to the outside world today has been through the nurses. They are all terrific. The morning guy wanted to talk politics, and as long as there is a fair amount of agreement, I never mind doing that. He also knew one of the two people whom I know who went through this here (eight years ago) and was pleased to hear that I had been in contact. The midday woman has a hugely sympathetic heart. For a while yesterday, she just stood by me, smiling behind the mask. It made me a little uncomfortable at first, until I realized she was just being with me. It didn't matter if we spoke. After that, I was completely won over. Today, she told me the dizziness is caused by the anticonvulsant. A little dizziness beats a seizure. That's for sure.

She also knows the two people whom I know who had treatment here and are now thriving. We talked about how people react so differently to very similar treatments. These two both had *leukaemia*, not *myelofibrosis*, and at least one had chemo before the transplant and was severely weakened. One was in and out in only three weeks! The other had a really rough time of it and the prospects were not so clear for a while. I'd be happy for something in between! The night nurse I see less often. But she also has been warm, attentive, and caring. And she gave me a sleeping pill to take later.

The transplant doctor checked in. She expressed concern about my kidneys in relation to the optional fourth day of chemo. She wants to see what my readings look like on Monday before deciding whether to give me the fourth day. This is one of those difficult decisions that come up in treatment. A fourth day could possibly really foul up my kidneys, rendering me temporarily or permanently dialysis dependent. However, it would improve the prospects for the success of the transplant. But she stressed that she has done it successfully with just three days of chemo.

From what I hear from my outside sources and the second nurse, on Monday, after three days of chemotherapy, when the weekly nursing staff returns, I can expect to be feeling at least weaker - maybe worse still. Apparently, I need to get all my partying in this weekend! Those who know me well know that I did not feel particularly ill when entering the hospital. Except for a few random days when I could not drag myself off the couch because I was so fatigued, I have felt like I have been running at about 90 percent of my full energy level. Full enough for no one to notice, unless they already knew. That, I am told, is all about to come crashing down.

8
Day 5: Vegetarianism Is Not an Option

Today, the doctors introduced a new medicine called *anti-thymocyte globulin* (ATG). It's an infusion harvested from rabbits that have been pumped up to produce antibodies that can destroy human T-cells. The ATG will serve as a prophylactic against the rejection of the new stem cells.

I have no idea how the rabbits are treated. I imagine that they are at least encaged. I don't know what the over-production of antibodies does to them. I assume that bunny suffering is involved in making this treatment possible for me.

What is my responsibility for their suffering? It has already occurred and was not occasioned by my illness in particular. Does this free me to use the medicine without being implicated in the suffering? Some people who call themselves *roadkill vegetarians* accept an argument like that across the board. In bumper sticker form, if it's already dead, it's ok to eat. But it's not so easy to see what is at all vegetarian about that view. Nothing at my grocery store is ruled out. If one is opposed to unnecessary animal suffering, the reason not to eat meat is not due to the animals that suffered in producing what you are eating, but due to contributing to the demand for meat that causes other animals to suffer. By analogy then, by using this medicine, perhaps I am contributing to the demand that will cause rabbits to suffer from the production of the drug. That contribution might be real, but it's very small.

How should I think about this? It's far from clear that there would be *any* market effect if I did not use the medication. No reduced demand. Markets are complicated, and I don't understand them very well, but economists say that they tend to adjust. My usage might simply be 'corrected for' by someone else. But then maybe the issue is not whether my usage makes a discernible difference causally to the well-being of any particular bunny; maybe simply being involved in the structural process that causes suffering to rabbits is something that requires a moral justification, something more than 'I want to save my own skin.'

Imagine some rabbits are hooked up to a machine that shocks them if a crank is turned often and fast enough. Some of our actions cause the crank to turn, actions like eating rabbit meat and using medicines derived from rabbits. Any person who eats rabbit meat regularly contributes far more to the turning of the crank than someone who only once uses the medicine. Moreover, avoiding eating rabbit meat (or any other kind of meat) can be done at no great loss for most people, but for those who need the ATG for a successful transplant, avoiding its use could be deadly. I would like to say that these two reasons excuse the use of ATG. Someone else will have to decide if that's rationalizing.

The infusion of ATG runs over the course of three days, with today being the longest at thirteen hours. So, in addition to the bags of water and the two kinds of chemo, Ginger Rogers is especially loaded down today. Hope she can still dance! The truth is that I'm feeling a little tired today and may not be dancing that much myself.

I woke up early and did my exercises, 30 minutes on the bike and fifteen minutes with the dumbbells. I took a little nap after breakfast and have been light-headed and tired ever since. Otherwise, I am doing fine. I'm looking forward to seeing my wife and son later today. But I will be spending lots of time in bed, the place the nurses want me to be anyway when receiving the ATG. In different circumstances, this would be a bit of a vacation.

Spare a thought or a prayer of gratitude for the bunnies.

9

Day 4: Sweatin' and Shakin'

Last night, the rabbit antibodies disagreed with me. Around 6 p.m., I started to shiver; then it turned to the sweats. The fever burned, and the elevated blood pressure pounded most of the night. Apparently, there's nothing particularly unusual about my experience. But knowledge of that didn't make it feel any better.

The evening nurse scolded me for letting several cables drop to the floor when I got up to use the toilet. I couldn't tell if she was serious or somehow playing. But I consoled myself with the thought that perhaps every hospital has a Nurse Ratched. The nighttime nurse was attentive and comforting, but clearly also a force to be reckoned with. These two are veterans of the transplant ward. They've seen it all. They know how to make sure what needs to be done - medicine taken, rest taken - gets done, but they also have sympathy for the patients. One part drill sergeant, another part camp counsellor. For the evening shift, the nurse mix tends towards the drill sergeant.

It was a fitful night. The fever and sweats lasted nearly throughout. I awoke feeling better, but distinctly worse than yesterday morning and the day before. The baseline is dropping along with my blood counts. The chemo seems to be effective in killing off blood production. My haemoglobin is down, which results in fatigue. I didn't exercise this morning. It was just too damn hard after the night I'd had. I didn't take the decision lightly. I know it's important to do. If tonight goes better, I'll do it tomorrow.

My mouth is as dry as a desert. This brings no joy to eating. The bread and cheese for breakfast felt like wadded-up paper in my mouth. It was all I could do to swallow it. That's also the chemo.

I'm getting more rabbit antibodies today (and tomorrow). The nurses tell me it should not be as bad as yesterday. In any case, my big plans for the day are to spend it mostly in bed, dozing and waiting for it to pass.

10 Day 3: Making Decisions When You Can't Think

'Draw a square with three straight lines,' the janitor said to me. I looked up from the paper at him and thought to myself, I'm not sure I have the energy to do this. 'Don't overthink it!' You're talking to the wrong guy, buddy! 'And no, you can't use the side of the sheet of paper as an extra line.' My head felt packed with cotton wool. I wasn't really enjoying the challenge. In reality, I could barely even under-think the problem. When he wrote an answer, □ | | |, all I felt was tired. Next puzzle:

> Suppose you got a wolf, a sheep, and a lettuce on one the side of the river, and you need to transport them across to the other side. You can only take one at a time, boat's not big enough for more. But you can't leave the wolf alone with the sheep; the sheep will be eaten. And you can't leave the sheep

> alone with the lettuce, or the lettuce be eaten. How do you get them across?

I couldn't get any farther than taking the sheep across first. I was mad about that because, unlike the first puzzle, this one was no trick. I blamed the cotton wool in my head.

My wife is a breast cancer survivor. During treatment, she received chemotherapy once every three weeks for four or five months. She used to speak of 'chemo brain', a generalized lack of sharpness. I think it's descending on me, and I think the janitor knows. Don't let me make any bets with him!

When my son came to visit, I presented both puzzles to him. He also gave up on the square and three lines one, and he was not happy about the right answer. But he cranked out the answer to the river crossing. It goes like this: first, take the sheep across. Next, go back with an empty boat; grab the wolf and deposit it on the other side. But before crossing back, grab the sheep; cross back with it; leave the sheep; but grab the lettuce. Go back across with the lettuce; leave it over there with the wolf. Finally, go to the original side with an empty boat; pick up the sheep; and bring him to the other side. My son might have a career in logistics or maybe directing.

Yesterday evening and last night were thankfully considerably better than the night before. But even though I slept reasonably well, I noticed this morning that it takes me a long time to get going in the morning. I did finally get to my exercise routine and take my shower, just before the nurse came in to put a bag of *fludarabine* on Ginger Rogers and hook me up.

The question of what to do about my kidneys and chemotherapy was solved by compromise. You might recall that the doctor spoke of a trade-off between the possibility of the fourth day of chemo damaging my weakened kidneys, rendering me dialysis-dependent, and receiving only three days of chemo, as typically people over 60 do, which would make the transplant itself a bit riskier. She recommended splitting the difference. So, on this day, the fourth day of chemotherapy, I received only the *fludarabine* and not the *busulfan*. She has done it this way before with success, and she seemed confident. Who am I to know better?

As patients, we put ourselves in the trust of doctors. We make ourselves vulnerable to their judgements. It's not that we have no role to play at all. For how we want to live is at stake. But we can't pretend to have a better grasp of the empirics than the doctors.

I'm fuzzy in the head, dizzy when I stand up, and tired most of the time. I'm hardly a model decision-maker right now. Two things stand out about that short discussion and decision regarding chemotherapy. First, insofar as she is recommending a slight reduction of chemo on behalf of my kidneys, she must be confident that the reduction does not change the likelihood of success all that much. Why do something on behalf of my kidneys if I'll be dead? Second, when I first spoke to her early last summer, she seemed eager to point out the risks of a transplant and unwilling to recommend any decision at all. She adopted the position of informing, not advising. Just now, her stance was firm. She must feel strongly about it.

Being a patient is not only about being patient. There's a boatload of trust involved, too.

11

Day 2: Nausea and Fatigue

Yesterday afternoon and evening were comparatively good stretches. The last bag of chemo went empty with little fanfare. No marching bands were to be seen on the transplant ward. But I felt almost ready to join one. I had plenty of energy and even felt about 80 percent of my normal self all evening. I slept for a very long time last night, but this morning, I experienced the familiar feeling of not being able to get started. The nurses woke me at 7 a.m. to hook me up to an IV of antibiotics. After the IV, I was requested to shower while my bed was changed. It was in a heavy morning fog that I went into the shower. I know people for whom that is usual, but it never has been for me, and I found it disconcerting. Breakfast was delivered and I could hardly face it. I forced down the yogurt, juice, and kiwi, but I refused the arid roll. The meal that is delivered to me seems to overlap about 75 percent with what I order. There's always an element of surprise involved.

After breakfast, the nurse always cleans the valves on the tubes of my catheter. Today, that meant I could lie back down, which was welcome. Nausea seemed to be visiting me, really for the first time. And it was a pretty dispiriting feeling. Because the catheter goes in at my neck, the four tubes that it divides into hang high on my shoulders. I can't see very well what she does, but she seems to attend to the dressing, sanitizing things, and checking for blockages. She's talkative, and I like her. Recently, she moved to this transplant clinic from another one so that she could move in with her boyfriend. They are remodelling his grandma's old house together. I started to drift through the story. When she was finished, she declared that I had about twenty minutes before she would hook me up to a bag full of rabbit antibodies.

So, with a huge heave and a tremendous act of will, I mounted the stationary bicycle. It was the last thing I felt like doing, really. But I have been scared by nurses' stories - they are so devious - of people who nearly waste away in here after five to six weeks of doing nothing. A sports consultant also came by yesterday and stressed the importance of keeping active. I got sixteen minutes of riding in before the nurse came back with a bag to connect me to. I was managing to ride but not having any fun due to the tremendous headwind of chemo and little voices in my head calling me back to bed. I was glad to quit when the nurse came back in. I hadn't lost, but

I also hadn't won. I resolved that I'd finish up the riding and hit the dumbbells later on today.

After she hooked me up to the rabbit antibodies, I laid back down. I drifted in bed until lunch. The meal consisted of some sort of white fish and boiled potatoes with white sauce and a side of zucchini delicately brought to the consistency of jarred baby food. I ate it with an enthusiasm that surprised me. Afterwards, I felt a return of energy.

The energy ebbs and flows are frustrating. I've learned to act when I can, and simply to wait it out when I can't do much of anything else. Will it be like this after the transplant on Thursday, or am I in for something completely different? I suspect the latter. The nurses tell me that everyone reacts differently. With the mission of destruction over, it will be the beginning of the critical rebuilding mission. I don't know how long the chemo and rabbit anti-bodies linger, but I imagine my travails will be very different after the transplant, waiting and hoping for the successful rebuilding of an immune system that will protect me - waiting for my cure.

12

Day 1: Courage

It's Wednesday. Last Thursday, feeling reasonably healthy, I checked into the stem cell transplant unit. I did that completely voluntarily in the hopes of curing a disease that would otherwise kill me in the coming few years. A week ago, I could easily run several miles, lift weights for a good half an hour, do work-related tasks, and make meals for my family. I've had good care here. I'm in excellent hands. Yet, when I got up out of bed to shower this morning, I was so weakened that I thought I might black out in the shower stall. The doctor was not surprised to hear this. He recommended using the shower stool they provide. That's why it's there. He explained that as a result of the chemotherapy, my haemoglobin has dropped so low that I am very weak. When I stand up and go into a warm shower, I have a low blood pressure moment, and blackout is a possibility. I guess it's all routine. I had no idea what the routine was when I checked in last week. I still really don't. And I guess it varies a fair bit from person to person. But I've become astonishingly weak, very quickly. I've never read a first-person account of stem cell transplants. I could find nothing on the internet to prepare myself. Now I wonder if there is a secret confederacy of patients, dedicated to not telling others how crappy it gets, in order not to scare people away from having the life-saving procedures.

Tomorrow is transplant day, soon after which I hope the pendulum swings from destruction to rebuilding. If I were to walk out of this hospital today, I would not get far. Before long, I'd succumb to fatigue, and without much of a working immune system, I would probably catch a severe infection. The bodily processes that make up this living organism that I would go into a deep crisis. I have no choice but to move forward with the transplant. It's the only option, but it was also the best option when I chose it. I do have a choice, however, regarding how I face the travails and risks that are ahead.

Aristotle thought that courage was the virtue that is particularly called upon when facing fear, and the fear of death in particular (2009: III.6). Courage is not only a martial virtue, but also has particular application in battle. Like all virtues of character, Aristotle thought it was concerned with feeling and acting, neither too much nor too little but the right amount, in the right way, and at the right time - a mean between extremes. The courageous person is neither fearless nor a coward, but feels the fear that is appropriate and acts accordingly in the face of it. Aristotle claimed that we come to have the virtues of character, courage included, by imitation. If at first, we have to quell an excessive level of fear in order to act in a way a courageous person would, over time so acting may produce results. If at first, we have moral imposter syndrome when acting courageous, over time we simply become courageous.

Curiously, Aristotle did not think of courage in relation to facing the dangers that manifest as a result of ill health. Perhaps there was little role for courage, given the health practices of his time, but there certainly is now. Aristotle thought that the virtues were only applicable where one has the capacity for choice. No one chooses to be sick. And once sick, in his time, there were few choices regarding care, or how best to live with illness. In Atul Gawande's insightful book, *Being Mortal: Death and What Matters in the End*, he writes that

> For all but our most recent history, death was common, an ever-present possibility. It didn't matter whether you were five or fifty. Every day was a role of the dice ... Life and health would putter along nicely, not a problem in the world, then illness would hit and the bottom would drop out like a trapdoor.
>
> (2014: 36)

People did not linger in death, and they did not live for long periods of time with serious chronic illness. How to live in the face of a serious disease, how to face the risks of medical treatments, and how to prepare for one's steady decline are not perennial questions, because medical care didn't provide a context in which such concerns arose. But with advances in medical care, these are important questions for us.

Patience seems particularly appropriate in regard to waiting - for a diagnosis, for the test results to arrive, for a therapy to show some effect, or for some counts to improve. Patience counsels the continued enjoyment of the value that life offers, the value that anxiety about the future eats away. Patience is needed in the face of imagined risks. It's tempting to think that courage is needed in the face of real ones. The idea would be that both patience and courage direct us to the continued pursuit of the value that remains in life in the face of fears that could overwhelm us and prevent us from the full appreciation of that value. Courage, however, is typically thought of as important when we have a choice to do something dangerous and fear might discourage it. Courage carries us through. But once one is in transplant protocol, there is not really a choice, courage doesn't seem quite applicable. Still, it helps if we can keep our fears checked, and for lack of a better term, perhaps we should just call the capacity to do that 'courage'.

13 Day 0: Communion

Transplant day started earlier than usual. The night nurse came in at 5 a.m. to draw blood and to give me a preparatory infusion. I was too groggy at the time to remember now if it was an antibiotic or an immune system suppressant or something else. I was awoken again shortly after 7 a.m. with more preparations. I was hooked up to a big bag of immunosuppressants and to a smaller one of water. I sat at my desk for a while and then the transplant doctor came in. She told me the plan. The transplant would happen in the morning. Enough stem cells had been harvested yesterday to do the transplant before noon. There were not enough to freeze extras should they be needed, but the donor would be available for more in that event.

My blood counts suggest that the chemo had achieved the intended effect. I have entered into *aplasia*. This is the condition in which one has no self-generating immune system. My white counts have nearly hit the bottom. The platelet counts are the lowest ever. And I have anaemia like never before. I used the stool this morning when showering. I'll remain transfusion-dependent now for at least two weeks.

The anonymous donor provided the stem cells yesterday. He's 32 years old and from a large city in the east. He is a perfect match. He even has the same blood type. I don't know any more about him. I wonder what conviction led him to help. Why was he so generous with his time and body? Perhaps he's a member of a helping profession, and donating is part of the professional culture. Maybe a fireman. Maybe it's done out of religious faith. Or maybe there is a family history of a similar illness. I've never known anyone who has donated stem cells. Plenty of people donate blood, especially at colleges and universities. I have even done that. But donating stem cells is less common. I can imagine that with stem cell donation there is a deeper sense of satisfaction. The donor is *the* person making the life-saving effort possible, not just one of many donors contributing to the cause.

Whatever his reason for helping, it was with a deep sense of gratitude that I accepted his communion gift this morning at about 10.50 a.m. I was connected to a bag of his stem cells; some 5.4 million, I'm told. The tube flowed red for about an hour. But I was also hooked up to some kind of anti-allergen infusion, which made me drowsy. So, I drifted in and out of a sleep as sweet as frankincense.

Now I wait, once again. The stem cells need to graft and then begin the formation of the new marrow. The hope is to find evidence of the pump being primed, in the form of rising blood counts, in two weeks. Risk of infection will be the main threat during that time. After that, we hope that the new immune system takes its guard dog duty seriously and attacks only hostile outsiders.

I know the process is not over yet. But I feel a little lighter today. Whatever else, that disease is past. So, say a toast tonight for the demise of a disease, and for further health! I'd like nothing more than to join in, but on this ward tonight I get nothing stronger than the words of T.S. Eliot: '[T]o make an end is to make a beginning. The end is where we start from' (1943: n.pag.).

14 Day +1: Confinement

There's little to report on the first day with the new stem cells floating around inside. The transfusion raised my counts above the scarily low level. Gone is the vague bad taste in my mouth and the fuzzy head of chemo. Fatigue and mild nausea unfortunately remain powerful forces pulling me to bed today. I did get my exercise routine in, but I may have overdone it. I feel like I've run a marathon. Well, I don't actually know what that feels like. But I am exhausted. My appetite is not very strong, but maybe the food here has something to do with that.

I have developed strong aversions. After the chemo, I haven't been able to face the two bags of potato chips that my wife brought me. So much so that I had to put them away in the closet. I can't drink sparkling water anymore. And worse yet, one of the two mouthwashes I am required to use four times a day is disgusting to me.

I also, for the first time, felt confined today, really confined. After only a week in this room, I feel like busting out. Don't worry - lack of energy keeps me from doing anything stupid. The janitor told me that when patients' counts are high enough for them to walk in the halls, they are allowed to go to a little window and breathe the fresh air through their masks. Oh, how I dream of that window!

15

Day +2: Waiting and Anxiety

I'm doing as well as I could hope for physically. No serious side effects of the transplant have arisen yet. And so far, there are no indications of serious infections. And I had more energy and less nausea today than yesterday. Currently, the main issue is that I still have little appetite and eating feels like a chore.

Waiting for the next two to three weeks to see if the stem cell graft and begin producing blood is going to be much harder for me than waiting for the transplant itself. Pre-transplant I was happily at home with my family playing an enthusiastic role in the family, running in the woods with Rex, and working. Surrounded by those whom I love and engaged in meaningful work, my life was full of valuable roles and activities. The Horace-Jesus-Epictetus attitude (that I spoke about in Chapter 3) was easier to attain and maintain pre-transplant because it encouraged my attention on those activities. And it fed on itself; the more I enjoyed them, the easier it was not to be distracted by worry. But now I am isolated from all that. I am now living alone. Well almost, the healthcare providers are always good for an interruption. The repeated measurements of my temperature, weight, and blood pressure, the daily blood drawing, and the many IVs are constant reminders that my circumstance is still precarious and uncertain. And everyday life is far less rewarding. It's lonelier. It's boring. And it's antiseptic. When my wife visited, we sat and held hands, hers in a plastic glove, while watching *Ghostbusters*.

The carpe diem attitude seems to have limited force in these circumstances, because there is so little in *diem* to want to *carpe*. Debilitating worry is, of course, still irrational in the sense that it only undermines whatever good could come out of the present circumstances. That provides some leverage on the worry. But on its own, it's not much. Right now, I need as much contact as I can get with friends and family, either physically or virtually. Light diversions help too, especially when I'm too tired for anything else. A little work helps in connecting me with activities that are important to me. And after last night, I've embraced the utility of a sleeping pill.

These next few weeks, I think, are not going to be easy. But they'll be easier if I continue to feel relatively good physically, if the side effects and infections remain minimal. If all goes as is likely, we will be able to celebrate the blood production beginning before too long.

Writing helps as well. It gives me something to focus on.

16
Day +3: Relaxed

Whereas the first two days after the transplant were a difficult period of readjustment to further waiting, today was a good day. Lovely and sunny outside my window. I awoke feeling fine. My energy was slightly less than the day before, and that proved to be due to lower haemoglobin levels. The doctor decided it was time for another transfusion. Now with two new bags of blood, I'm gassed and ready to roll for a couple of days.

The doctor's visit was very encouraging. It's far too early to tell if anything is going on in the rebuilding department, but he was happy with how stable things are and with the lack of complications thus far. That, he thought, bodes well.

I did a slightly lighter-than-usual exercise routine and then committed myself fully to being in recovery mode. This was the first day since entering the hospital that I felt so completely relaxed. It was a treat! In the afternoon, my family came for a visit, and we watched most of *The Blues Brothers* together. The two of them were sitting with gowns and masks on and me lounging in between. It would have made for quite a family picture, 'Greetings from the Transplant Unit!'

17 Day +4: Toiling and Spinning

A friend reminded me of the passage in Matthew that precedes the one that I quoted in Chapter 3. Matthew 6:28-29: 'Consider the lilies of the field, how they grow; they toil not, neither do they spin: and yet I say unto you, that even Solomon in all his glory was not arrayed like one of these' (1987). I have long loved that passage as an expression of wonder regarding nature and natural processes. The friend suggested that I consider the stem cells growing, neither toiling nor spinning, in their new home inside my bones. It is a wondrous thought! I marvel at how these things must work - not that I really understand them. In any case, I don't think that scientifically understanding how seed germination works, when it works, makes it any less wondrous that it works. In many cases, as is often the case with art, understanding can foster even greater appreciation. If all natural processes were one day well understood, we still have reason to sit back and marvel over their workings, over the comprehensibility of the whole, and, of course, over the sheer fact that something exists rather than nothing. There is something wondrous about those stem cells growing (I hope!) deep inside my bones.

Two events from the day: this afternoon, I was visited by a pair of third-year medical students, making the rounds for their studies. These were two young women who until then had never examined a living human body! Their job was to knock around on my belly, listen with a stethoscope, and examine my lymph nodes. They were nervous, hesitant, and self-conscious. It was all very sweet. I did what I could to put them at ease. After all, I am happy to further the cause of advancing medical studies!

The oncological psychotherapist also paid me a visit today. We talked at some length about the experience of being a patient. She talks about the almost total loss of autonomy that one experiences when entering a hospital. Before one enters the hospital, one is busy dealing with the disease alongside everything else. But in the hospital, treatment of the disease rules, and one's life is governed by the protocol for responding to the disease. So, when one is thrown into the waiting mode, without an everyday life to participate in, it is a much more foundation-shaking experience. Without our usual everyday projects, we more easily feel at a loss. And the realization that one is sick, indeed very sick, can produce a profound loss of orientation, a vertigo. All of these points to the importance of maintaining a routine of valuable activities, things that are meaningful, and more than just waiting. Rebuilding life as the stem cells rebuild the immune system.

I remarked to her that I was less bothered at night after taking the pill the doctors prescribed several days ago. She informed me that it had nothing to do with the pills. Those take a couple of weeks to begin working. Life rebuilding, it seems, has already begun. I'd like to think the same is true of the stem cells, neither toiling nor spinning.

It was another beautiful day here, and a good one for me.

18 Day +5: Healthcare for All Pt. 2

I am sitting in my hospital room in a bone marrow transplant unit in Frankfurt, Germany. I am a patient who has recently received a stem cell transplant. I am a US citizen, but I am a resident of a country that has a health insurance system funded by payroll taxes. Participation is mandatory. That insurance program covers 90 percent of the population; high earners can opt out by purchasing private insurance. But for the vast majority, they pay a tax of about 7.3 percent of their earnings, which are matched by the employer. Government financing covers those who are unemployed or unable to work. The insurance is administered by one of several non-profit organizations that differ very little in coverage benefits because of the mandatory high level of minimum coverage. So, nearly everyone receives essentially the same coverage. We are able to choose the insurer we want from among these non-profits, whose funding comes from the payroll taxes. If you think of these non-profits as the insurers, the government is their re-insurer. Doctors and pharmacists in private practice are reimbursed by these insurers.

I am not yet a permanent resident of this country. I live here legally on a temporary work visa. Nonetheless, I am a full participant in the insurance plan. The costs of stem cell transplants vary considerably, but in the United States, they average about $800.000. Here, where the majority are not covered by for-profit insurance, transplants average a bit more than $250.000. In my case, that is what I expect the insurance plan will end up paying for my transplant. When I walk out of the hospital, my bill will be a 10€ per-day charge. This is not because I have a Platinum plan at a cost affordable only for the jet-setting global professoriate. On the contrary, I am getting the same coverage for the same excellent treatment that anyone else living here would receive. That's what healthcare for all has meant to me and my family.

Today, the doctor paid me a visit and handed me a letter that I need to submit to the insurance administrator. The letter states that when I am released, I will need to make frequent follow-up visits at a time when my immune system will be weak. By the doctor's orders, I am not allowed to take public transportation. In this case, the insurance is required to reimburse my taxi fare. Once again, a standard benefit of this single-payer scheme.

When Paul Ryan sought to defend a Republican healthcare plan offered to Congress, a plan which according to an independent analysis of the Congressional Budget Office would render 14 million people uninsured within the first year, he leaned in on the rhetoric of liberty. This is because he couldn't plausibly claim that the plan would be good for health outcomes. He said,

> If the government says, 'Thou shalt buy our health insurance,' the government estimates are going to say people will comply. And when you replace that with, 'We're going to have a free market and you buy what you want to buy,' they're going to say not nearly as many people are going to do that.
>
> (Ryan 2017: n.pag.)

There are costs to the kind of liberty that the Republicans were advocating. The basic principle of insurance is risk-pooling. If people participate voluntarily on the basis of their beliefs about their own risks, participation will be limited mostly to those who see themselves as vulnerable (the poor, the sick, and the elderly) and the premiums will be expensive. Universal coverage not only broadens coverage, but it also reduces premiums.

Americans already pay more for healthcare than their counterparts in other wealthy countries. In

2013, the Commonwealth Fund conducted a study of health and healthcare in the wealthiest countries in the world, the OECD countries. It found that 'In 2013, the U.S. spent far more on health care than these other countries ... Despite spending more on health care, Americans had poor health outcomes, including shorter life expectancy and greater prevalence of chronic conditions.' Spending as a percentage of GDP in the United States is just over 17 percent. In continental Europe, it tends to be just over 11 percent. For the United Kingdom, it is just under 9 percent. More spending in the United States did not result in more doctors to serve the population. There are 2.6 physicians for every 1000 people in the United States, and 4.1 in Germany. More spending in the United States does not increase life expectancy. Life expectancy at birth in the United States is 78.8 years, and in Germany it's 80.9. Nor does more spending yield a healthier population. The percentage of the population over 65 with two or more chronic conditions in the United States is 68 and in Germany only 49. And the number of infant deaths per 1000 live births in the United States is 6.1 and in Germany it's nearly half that at 3.3 (The Commonwealth Fund 2015). In general, the coverage is far wider in Europe; the costs of care are lower, and health outcomes are better.

What about the liberty that Ryan invoked? Germany can hardly be described as a tyranny. Freedom of religion, speech, and movement are all secure.

Elections are free and far less corrupted by money than in the United States. Better health outcomes at lower costs have not been purchased at the cost of basic liberty. Yes, people must pay payroll taxes. But being secure in their healthcare coverage, they are also free of the worry that illness will wipe them out financially, or that they will be unable to pay for appropriate care. And perhaps the biggest difference is in the attitude of solidarity. It is simply unthinkable for most people here that a person should be left to suffer ill health or even death due to the lack of insurance. Ask not for whom the bell tolls.

When I am healthy enough to leave the hospital and go home, I will count myself as fortunate to be living here, where coverage and excellent care were made available by taxpayers. More than that, it *is* unthinkable to me that someone with my disease in the United States might fail to get the lifesaving transplant she needs because she is either uninsured or without the insurance that would cover the procedure. That outrage will cast a long shadow on my feeling of good fortune.

19
Day +6: Patience *and* Hope?

I am happy to share an important life lesson that I have learned over the course of my stay at the transplant unit: if you have to rinse your mouth several times a day with two different medicated mouth washes, one of which you find foul, repulsive, and dreadful, rinse with the bad one first. It would be too embarrassing to tell you how long it took me to figure out that doing it in that order helps to mitigate the lingering wretched taste.

The medication regimen imposed on me is impressive. Orally, I take fourteen different kinds of medications, most of these more than once a day. Additionally, through the IV, there flow various immunosuppressants, antibiotics, and hydration infusions. The medications tend to proliferate, as some are aimed at facilitating the success of the transplant and others deal with the side effects of the first kind of meds. For example, I take an immunosuppressant, which dials down the immune system so as to reduce the severity and incidence of battles between the emerging immune system and my organs. But the one that I take has the side effect of increasing blood pressure, which in my case was already slightly elevated. As a consequence, I had a couple of mornings this week when my systolic pressure (the top one of the two) was through the roof. Dealing with that requires taking another kind of medication. And all of this, of course, has a certain learn-by-doing character; every organism is different and differently complex. So, doses need to be adjusted to achieve the desired effect. But, of course, sometimes you can't just tweak one dosage because it has side effects that have to be managed. The doctors have a name for mixing multiple meds: Polypharmacy.

My homework every evening is to lay out all my pills in a tray with four compartments for the different times during the following day that I am supposed to take them. Not a day has gone by when the plan that I have followed has been the same as the previous day. In some cases, the milligrams of the actual medication differ from the milligrams on the plan, in which case I have to do the calculation and either halve or double the dosage. After the chemo, managing the polypharmacy has been taxing work. Sometimes it takes all my powers of concentration, and it can be exhausting! In frustration, I have grumbled to myself about this task being left to me to manage. Does the nursing staff just want to shove this task off on me? In a less quarrelsome mood, I suspect that it is some kind of competency test; when I was receiving chemo, the night nurse would check my work. And once or twice she playfully scolded me for screwing up. I think that when it comes time to release a patient, they need to be sure that the meds can be managed at home.

In an effort to reincorporate aspects of normal life into my life here, I'm meeting this evening with an internet book group. There are three core members of this group, and we have met off and on for over ten years, first in person when we all taught at the same university and after that virtually when two of us moved. We cover the fields of classics, political science, and philosophy. We pick a hard piece of philosophy that we are all at least somewhat interested in and we read it over the course of many months. We've read lots of different things, including Plato's *Statesman*, St. Augustine's *City of God*, Nietzsche's *The Gay Science*, and Adorno's *Minima Moralia*. For some time now, we've been reading volume one of Ernst Bloch's *The Principle of Hope.* I cherish this group and my friendship with the other members. It's wonderful to get back to meeting with them.

The section of Bloch that we are discussing tonight is relevant to my earlier invocation of Epictetus in Chapter 3. Epictetus's attitude of focusing on what is in one's control is a tonic against anxiety, but perhaps it also rules out more positive future-oriented attitudes about things that are uncertain, attitudes like hope. Bloch interprets ancient thought as sceptical about the value of hope due to the unhappiness that unfounded hope may cause. His major purpose in the book is to vindicate what he sees as the really fundamental importance of hope. In his conclusion of a discussion of ancient scepticism about hope, he says the following:

> And founded hope especially, that is, hope mediated with the real Possible, is so far removed from evil ... that it in fact represents the at least half-open door appearing to open on to pleasant objects, in a world which has not become a prison, which is not a prison.
>
> (Bloch 1995: 334)

20 Day +7: A Letter Arrives

Today marks two weeks that I have been in the hospital and one week since the transplant. I am feeling better than I expected to feel at this point. A bit tired today and I will probably need another couple of bags of red blood cells tomorrow or the next day. But that should keep me going for a while.

My white counts have hit rock bottom. With respect to infection, it's an especially risky time. But various stores of antibiotics stand ready to be tapped. I'm already taking some antibiotics, both prophylactically and in response to a gastrointestinal bug. Still, there could be a need for more. There is no rebuilding the new immune system without the counts bottoming out. So, this phase must be gone through. For patients who have had *leukaemia*, the average waiting time after the transplant before the first signs of rebuilding are measured is fourteen days. *Leukaemia* is not my disease. But although it is rare, it is less rare than *myelofibrosis.* A lot of the information one finds about stem cell transplants online is to do with *leukaemia* and not *myelofibrosis*. If the time to regeneration is roughly the same, maybe in a week there will be some signs.

I received a letter today from my donor, written the day after he donated the cells. It was strange and wonderful to receive. There is this person out there, whom I don't know; he has just rescued me, and now he is writing to me. He told me of his thoughts for my family and friends, how happy he was to help, and that I will never be alone. A gracious and beautiful gesture of compassion and support. I am speechless.

21 Day +8: Anaemia

Today has been low energy. All the counts are falling. That includes the haemoglobin; so I am very anaemic, leaving me lethargic. I did get in a very easy bike riding session. By doctor's orders, I can't break a sweat because my platelets are so low that bleeding in the head could result. That would mess up my plans. The nurses are very strict, even scolding, about this. When I got out of the shower, I dried myself with one of the coarse towels they provide – I've come to like the coarseness against my itchy dry skin. After that, when I put the industrial-strength moisturizer on my skin, I noticed that I was bleeding in two spots. Low platelets once again. Guess I need to go more lightly with the towel.

The day consisted mostly of resting, watching *The Office* (American version), and reading *Anna Karenina.* By the end of the day, my doctor decided to give me a platelet transfusion. So, they hoisted a bag of pale yellow-orange liquid that looked a bit like watered-down dahl and connected me to it via an IV. The doctor explained that this would allow more exercise tomorrow. But unless they also feed me a couple of bags of red cells, I might not feel much up to it.

22
Day +9: Why I Write

Strangely, I've had a little more energy today than yesterday, even though my haemoglobin is even lower. These energy levels are a mystery. The platelet transfusion yesterday increased my counts enough for a slightly more vigorous workout today. In addition to riding the bike at a very easy pace, I lifted the dumbbells a bit. The doctors held off with red blood cell transfusion for another day or two.

My tongue is swollen in my mouth, and it rubs against my teeth on the side, which is making the tongue sensitive. As a result of the chemo, slime production all throughout the gastrointestinal tract is way down, including the saliva in my mouth. The dryness of my mouth diminished the pleasure of my first room-delivered pizza last night. Still, it was great to get it. One big issue right now is dealing with my stressed-out kidneys. The chemo, as expected, has been hard on them. My potassium and creatinine levels are high; the former is a bigger concern than the latter. So, I am on diuretics that ensure that I get plenty of exercise walking to the toilet. I am also taking a substance that is supposed to capture the sodium in my gut before it metabolizes. The doctors expect the kidneys to bounce back to a better suboptimal level, and they don't seem terribly concerned yet.

When I return home, the house will need to be very clean because my immune system will still be weak. So, my wife hosted a house cleaning party today, promising pizza to everyone who showed up. Amazing, she tells me, over twenty people showed up! This is another example of the wonderful generosity that people are bestowing on us. The transplant itself, all of the words of support that I receive from friends, the friends who have come to help around the house, the neighbours who walk Rex, and now the house cleaners. It's all deeply moving. I am very grateful for it.

A friend wrote to me today asking if I sent upbeat messages so as not to worry people, and if that is the case urging me to be willing to show the hardship more. I started out writing with the purpose of informing family and friends. But the writing has taken on another kind of meaning for me. It has become a way in which I can make something out of the experience. It's not an experience that anyone would choose to have. As a patient, I may be hostage to the disease, the biochemistry, and the medical treatment. I may not be in control of the outcome, and I may have to suffer the experience. But if I have to suffer it, perhaps I can have something to show for it. This record itself is what I made of the experience, and I hope what I made is good. So, I work to convey the experience. The writing is not a therapy journal written only for myself. I would like it to be good in the sense that it touches others, but also in the sense that it is honest.

Honesty and comprehensiveness are not the same thing. I don't have to write about everything, but if I write about it, I aim to convey it honestly. If I'm not fully comprehensive, it's not because I am consciously choosing to avoid the bad stuff to spare the worry of my readers. I have talked a lot about the physical suffering. But so far, that has not been as bad as I expected. Regarding the psychological suffering, I think I've explored some dark places. Day +2 goes there, as does, to a lesser extent, +4 and the Chapter 3. I admit that it is harder for me to write about the psychological suffering. I think it's harder because it feels more exposing. Still, I hope that I haven't been avoiding writing about it and that when I write about it, I capture it. All of the support that I have received has helped a lot. The feedback on the writing has been very important to me. I also write for support.

The lack of great physical suffering thus far and receiving great support has allowed me to stay fairly upbeat. But I have come to realize that, by disposition, I am also generally positive. I'm just lucky that way. It's probably due to good parenting and good genes, both of which were simply gifts, not in any way accomplishments of mine. If I am upbeat, it's been a matter of good fortune: lack of severe physical suffering, the loving support of others, and the gift of a positive disposition. All of them also have reasons to be grateful.

23
Day +10: Why I Dyed My Hair Blue

I woke to a canker sore that had exploded just below the inner lip at the front right side of my mouth and to a tongue that felt like it had been rubbed with sandpaper on the sides. And the top of my throat had also joined in the chorus of pain. Once I was finally awake, I also realized just how tired I was. That's more or less been my condition for the day.

I tried to ride the bike, but after fifteen minutes I started to feel dizzy and weak, so I stopped. I received a red blood cell transfusion today, so my energy should improve tomorrow.

The doctor tells me that the mouth pain is just part of the process. It often gets bad enough that patients go on a 24-hour morphine drip. I guess that's one way to relax, but I hope it doesn't come to that, as I imagine that it makes reading and writing more challenging. The mouth pain will remain, I'm told, until the immune system becomes strong enough to fight back. And I learned that the first evidence of white blood cell production for patients with *myelofibrosis* is typically about a week later than for patients with *leukaemia*. So, I shouldn't really expect signs of success until about day +21. Sadly, that's still a full ten days away.

I used to say that when men a half a generation older than me would retire, they would often grow ponytails as an expression of their freedom from professional norms, but that when I retire, I intend to dye my hair blue. Shortly before entering the hospital, I decided to go blue before I lost it all. So, for several days before I entered the hospital, I walked about town with neon blue hair. My son found this pretty embarrassing, but he tried to be tolerant of my eccentricities. The night before I was admitted to the hospital, I cut my hair very short. Two weeks of washing it with high-octane germ-killing soap in here turned the colour to marine green, and then finally mostly to the underlying bleached blonde. Now, however, the shedding has begun in earnest. This morning, my nurse informed me that tomorrow would probably be shearing day.

Dear friends arrived today all the way from Long Beach, California! They are here to play my normal role of house elf. They are following two other friends, one from North Carolina and another from Paris. All of them have come a long way at considerable expense to help out. How very generous and sweet!

24 Day +11: Shorn

The shape of my day here seems pretty well-established. At 5 a.m., a nurse comes in and draws blood. They like to have the counts early so that they can adjust my medicine dosage for the day in response to the lab report. I then fall back to sleep and am roused at 7 a.m., at which point the first of many daily measures is taken. Blood pressure, temperature, pulse, and weight. I've been having trouble retaining weight due to diarrhoea caused by a gastrointestinal bug. The day before yesterday, I was down over seven pounds from my weight at entry. But we may be winning the battle against the bug, and I'm now only two pounds away from my entry weight.

After the measurements, the first of three morning infusions starts. I try to fit in 20–30 minutes of cycling and fifteen minutes of dumb bell work next, just before breakfast. The infusions are usually over by breakfast or by the end of breakfast. Then I am untethered from Ginger Rogers for a while. I chat with the janitor while he cleans the room. And then, while the nurse or orderly makes my bed, I take a shower. Today, the nurse shaved my head first. With my earring, I now look like the mascot for an American cleaning product, Mr. Clean; Meister Proper, I think he's called in Germany. I'd like to think that with my glasses on, the resemblance is more to Michel Foucault. Come to think of it, I have to wonder if Michel Foucault modelled himself after Mr. Clean?

After the shower, I lie on the bed while the nurse changes the dressing around my catheter. That's a process that lasts fifteen to twenty minutes. When that's all done, it's nearly 10.30 or 11 a.m., at which point I either respond to emails, read, or nap. In the last few days, napping has prevailed. Lying on the bed while the dressing is changed tends to induce a nap. The doctor visits once a day, and it's often during this time.

Lunch comes at noon. And there is more measuring of temperature, blood pressure, and pulse. In the afternoons, I'm untethered, and I do some combination of reading, watching TV, and journal writing. This is usually the high point of my energy for the day. Once a week, the sports trainer or the oncological psychotherapist pops in and we talk. After dinner, temperature, blood pressure, pulse, and weight measurements are taken again, and there are more infusions for an hour or so. In the evening, I have to organize my medication for the following day. After doing that, it's some combination of reading, watching TV, listening to music, and writing. Before going to bed, I get one or two more short infusions and sometimes a shot in the stomach. The lights go out at some point between 9 and 10 p.m. The night nurse checks on me periodically throughout the night. And then the drill starts again at 5 a.m.

25

Day +12: Tired, Itchy, and Hiccupping

Haemoglobin is one of the components of red blood cells. It has the important role of transporting oxygen, which is why people who are anaemic experience fatigue. In adult men, the normal range for haemoglobin is 13.5–17.5 g/dl and in women it's 12–16 g/dl. For several years, I have lived with haemoglobin counts in the 10s, which is classified as mild anaemia. I used to say that I simply lived at a higher altitude than everyone else. The fall in my counts had been gradual over several years - an early indication of *myelofibrosis* - and it didn't affect my life in any significant way. Exercise and a busy lifestyle were still possible. More than that, I had the benefit of a convenient excuse to offer my family, should I fall asleep while watching a movie! Before being admitted to the hospital, my haemoglobin count was in the 8–9 g/dl range, which is moderate anaemia. On Sunday, my count had fallen to 6.8 g/dl, severe anaemia. The transfusion later that day resulted in a count yesterday of 7.8 g/dl, still severe but much easier to handle. That gave me enough energy to both ride the bike and lift weights. Today, the count had fallen to 7.2 g/dl. And all I could muster was fifteen minutes on the bike. I will probably have another red blood cell transfusion tomorrow.

I have read that one symptom occasionally experienced by people with anaemia is pica, the urge to eat unusual things, like ice, clay, cardboard, crunchy foods, or raw starch. Fortunately, I have never had that! But I find that when my counts fall into the 8s, I am more easily cold. So, I've been chilly and fatigued today. It's just the afternoon, and I've already taken two naps, under the covers, of nearly an hour each.

The fatigue is augmented, I think, by an antihistamine that I took to deal with itchiness. It's not clear whether I'm itchy as a side effect of one of the many medications I take or as a result of the chemo-induced dry skin. But the sensation has gotten progressively worse. Strangely, there is no rash, just the itchy feeling on my forearms, shoulders, back, chest, and ankles. I think that I have a fairly high pain threshold, but my itchy threshold is low! I can't hold out long without scratching. And as amazingly satisfying as a good scratch can be to a persistent itch, it of course doesn't have a lasting effect. As soon as the scratching stops, the itch is back, sometimes even stronger. The cycle can be vicious. The scratching itself becomes a problem; the skin gets red and then raw. In the *Gorgias*, Socrates asks Callicles whether a person who has an itch and wants to scratch it can pass life happily simply by scratching (Plato 1967: 494c). I'm here to testify that one most certainly cannot.

During the day, it's easier to get distracted by other things and not notice the pin-pricking itchiness. But at night in bed, it's much harder. I woke up this morning with red patches on my right arm, presumably due to nighttime scratching. So, today the nurse prescribed an antihistamine, which, I think, might be making me especially sleepy today.

The last three or so days, I have been suffering from another odd and unexplained side effect. The hiccups. I hate the hiccups almost as much as I hate being itchy! These are severe enough to incapacitate me when they are especially intense. They come in waves, and it feels like the release of gastric pressure in my lower throat and upper gut. Sometimes, they are strong enough to hurt mildly. And every now and then, they also trigger additional pain in my sore throat. But on the whole, they are much more a nuisance than a cause of pain. The doctor tells me that they are not uncommon in patients in the transplant ward, but that they do not know what causes them. There is some medication that I can take that should help. I plan on doing that. I have no intention of being a hiccup hero.

It could be worse. The pain is not bad. I don't have a fever. And I don't have nausea or diarrhoea today. I'm not miserable really, just annoyed and uncomfortable.

The oncological psychotherapist just stopped by with ice cream bars. The simple pleasures! This is going to be a good evening!

26

Day +13: Waiting

I was chilly and tired again today. Chilly not due to a fever, thankfully, but, like the fatigue, due to the anaemia. I got in a record three naps. Everyone who has been urging me to take it easy should be very pleased! I don't take it easy very well. But the fatigue has been slamming me hard enough that I haven't really had a choice.

The doctor, a very tall young man, with glasses, and a brown beard under his surgical mask, paid me a visit. He said that everything looks to be on track. All that we can do presently is wait for the stem cells to graft and fight back the side effects that arise. My throat is very sore, which makes eating difficult. The itching is bearable with the antihistamine. And the fatigue just requires me to rest. I did do some reading for my Bloch reading group tonight. I also rode the bicycle for a mere fifteen minutes and had a nice visit with my wife at lunchtime.

27 Day +14: Signs of Progress

It's been three weeks since I entered the hospital and two weeks since the transplant. Almost as if in recognition of the milestone, the doctors and nurses delivered some fabulous news today. Neither spinning nor toiling, those stem cells seem to have set up residence and are beginning to grow blood cells! The doctor is not the type who would dance the jig with me, but that's what I felt like doing when she delivered the news. Instead, we both just smiled heartfelt smiles at each other.

The doctors watch two counts in particular, *leukocytes* and *neutrophils absolute*. *Leukocytes* make up the class of all white blood cells, and *neutrophils* are a particular kind of white blood cell that goes after bacteria and fungus. If you look at the Wikipedia page for white blood cells, you can see a cool picture of a *neutrophil* engulfing Anthrax bacteria. *Neutrophils* constitute 60–70 percent of all *leukocytes*. When your finger gets infected and pus forms, the pus is dead *neutrophils*. The *leukocytes* started climbing yesterday and the *neutrophils* today. I've received transfusions of red blood cells and platelets, but not of white blood cells. So, the best explanation seems to be that the immune system is regrowing. The doctor expects this to be a trend. And even mentioned that I might be free to go home later this week!

Fear of the graft not taking hold was my biggest anxiety after the transplant, even though the odds were good that it would. So, this comes as a huge relief. I do wonder if it could be a measurement error, or the process might halt. But the doctor didn't suggest either of these. So, I guess the possibilities must be remote.

In the expectation that my immune system will be stronger by next week, I was also moved to a double room today, which I have to myself now, but will share next Monday and perhaps beyond. It was strange leaving the other room. I won't say that I had become attached to it. But it was all that I knew for three weeks, and a lot happened there. Still, even walking down the hall to the new room with my gown and face mask on felt like a taste of freedom. Next stop, I hope, will be that window where I can smell the fresh air.

28
Day +15: Turn Me Loose, Set Me Free

I awoke in my spacious double room today. But I felt vaguely nauseous, chilly, and completely exhausted all day. I argued with myself about riding the bike, but finally dragged myself up on the saddle and rode for an easy fifteen minutes. I lay down for an hour or so after the morning routine was finished and then again after lunch, which I could barely eat. I spent most of the day in bed. Nobody is worried about this. The doctor has finally ordered a red blood cell transfusion, which I had thought for days that I'd be getting. After that, I should feel a bit better tomorrow.

The nurse who functions as a bit of a social worker and manages the release of patients from the unit came by. She's been kind and sympathetic throughout. When I checked into the unit, she said to me, 'I'll see you in three weeks.' Three weeks and a day later, she came by to talk to me about my release! She wasn't sure when - we'll follow the counts - but she mentioned that she was away the first three days of next week, so she needed to come by today in case I'm not here by the time she returns! During the conversation, I sat there marvelling that we were having a discussion about my release.

How will it be after I've been home for about six months, when life will be getting back to normal? I'd lived with the chronic disease for eighteen years until it morphed into a more serious one last year. Will I walk more lightly, free of the shadow of disease? Will the future seem more open-ended? I don't know, but I'm looking forward to finding out.

29
Day +16: Fresh Air

As I expected, I felt a great deal better today after yesterday's transfusion. All this vampire needs to keep running is a little blood.

I made it to that window today. Although it wasn't quite like the characters busting out in *Cuckoo's Nest*, it felt pretty damn good. The window is in a large kitchenette. The sky was blue, and up on the eleventh floor, the fresh wind gushed in. The window allows for a view in the opposite direction from the windows of my two rooms. I looked down over the brown-green river Main and out to the radiant skyscrapers on the other side. Light reflections shimmered busily off the buildings and were captured in the dull river. It's still early spring here, and trees have, for the most part, not yet budded. That permitted gazing far into the distance. Some ways away, I could see the town where I live. I wondered what friends and family were doing at that moment. On the river, there was plenty of commercial boat traffic, and along the river people were strolling with and without dogs. A workday for some and a rest day for others. I walked up and down the hall several times, but I kept coming back to that window, the cool, fresh air, and the warm, bright sunlight. Tomorrow, I might be allowed to go downstairs and out the doors.

Things are moving unbelievably quickly. Today, the doctor spoke of releasing me 'on vacation' on Monday afternoon, to go home for the night and then to return for the day on Tuesday, and then home again, finally that evening. This is all contingent on further growth in the counts, but all of a sudden, it seems to be upon us. It may all be too quick for my wife. She is concerned that the house is not yet sufficiently clean, and she is hobbled by a head cold that she doesn't want to transmit to me. So, I'll see what the doctors recommend tomorrow.

30 Day +17: Postponement

Another good day. The *leukocyte* and *neutrophil absolute* counts continue to rise steadily. Unfortunately, the latter was not quite high enough to allow me to go outside today. Maybe tomorrow. But there was dispiriting news today with respect to getting out tomorrow. My wife has a doctor's appointment in the morning, but the doctors here will not release me if she is contagious. So, ironically, I'll be spending my remaining days here rooting for her immune system, not mine. This was a big disappointment for me. But there is nothing else to be done.

My wife had another house cleaning party today. And again, the turnout was great! We are incredibly fortunate to have caring and helpful friends.

Part III
Recovery

31 Home Sweet Home

In the words of the great Jackie Gleason, 'How sweet it is!'

The short story is that the doctors decided the benefits of going home outweigh the risks. And apparently, those stem cells made surprisingly short work of it all. I'm home for the next 40 hours. If all goes well, I'll be officially discharged on Wednesday morning. However, the next six months will still be risky.

There's a lot that I want to write, but tonight is for hanging out with family and friends who have come a long way to help. More to come!

32
Home Update

After visiting the doctors today, they continued my 'vacation' till Friday, which is now my official check-out day. My counts continue to improve. My leukocytes are already in the normal range. Haemoglobin continues to rise. I'm only moderately anaemic. And the platelets lag behind but are also on the rise. None of this could have been predicted a week ago. It seems that I have some super-charged stem cells!

There's a lot I still would like to write, but honestly, I've just been too tired these last two days. Ordinary life, even in resting mode, is exhausting! How do healthy people do it all? My wife and I went for a 2-km walk along the river today while waiting for my blood results, and afterwards I needed to take a two-hour nap!

I am subject to a lot of rules to keep me on the road to recovery. My wife is keeping me on the straight and narrow. She even tattled to my doctor today that I mistakenly ate blueberries with my granola yesterday! (Thou shalt not eat fresh fruit that hasn't been peeled.) Imagine my humiliation!

33 The Social Determinants of My Survival

I've been thinking about the various circumstances that have worked in my favour.

Let's start with the global. I have benefited from living in a high-income country. According to the World Health Organization (WHO), residents of high-income countries get a life expectancy bonus of sixteen years in comparison to residents of low-income countries. The average life expectancy in low-income countries is just 60 years, while in high-income countries it is 76 years (WHO 2014: n.pag.). No doubt, many factors are at work there. Generally, early childhood health is much better in high-income countries and that has long-term effects. Even still, expensive and technologically complicated treatments, requiring a high degree of advanced training, such as stem cell transplants, are likely to be more readily available and more successful in high-income countries. A person living in, say, Malawi would be less likely to survive my illness.

I also live in a country in which it is considered a matter of justice that everyone is covered by medical insurance that provides for very high-quality treatment. A person living in the United States might be excluded from the life-saving treatment due to insurance that does not cover it, too high a co-payment, or lack of insurance altogether. Poor people covered by Medicaid and seniors covered by Medicare who suffer from *myelofibrosis* only became covered for a transplant in January of last year (UIC Today 2016). In other words, a person's access to life-saving treatment is far less secure in the United States.

I've benefited from being of European descent. It turns out that race (as a proxy for common ancestry) matters in finding a matched unrelated donor. Whether a potential donor is a match depends on genetics. People who share a common ancestry are more likely to be a match. There are over 40 million people registered around the world as possible donors, around half of them in the United States. Campaigns to register people in African and Asian countries have not taken off to a similar degree. And in the United States, the history of unjust medical 'experimentation' on African Americans is an obstacle to people's willingness to participate in registry efforts (Schmidt 2024). Additionally, people of African descent are by far the most genetically diverse group because of the long history of human movement out of Africa and into all the regions of the world. So, not only are there fewer donors of African descent, but also the genetic profile of a donor is also less likely to match the person in need (Nunes et al. 2020). I can only imagine the heartache of being denied access to a transplant because no donor can be found. I had a perfectly matched unrelated donor. Had I been of African descent, that would have been far less likely.

I've emphasized on several occasions how little success is a matter of a patient's own efforts and how much of it depends on the vagaries of complex biochemical processes, in particular the disease's response to therapy, as well as the skill and experience of the doctors and care staff. Survival is, in large part, a matter of good biochemical fortune. It's more like a gift than an accomplishment. But the language of 'gift' might suggest that it's just a matter of charity. The social determinants of survival are matters of policy. We survivors have had the good fortune not only of biochemistry but also of favourable social circumstances. That's an issue of justice. Better science can improve biochemical fortune across the board. Better politics can reduce health disparities.

34 Letting the Days Go By

I've been impressed with myself. With my abilities. In particular, my ability to sit around and do almost nothing at all. I didn't think I had it in me, really. As an adult, I have always been busy, very busy. The Protestant Work Ethic has featured prominently as part of my adult personality. (Mind you, my 16-year-old self was blissfully free of that.) But I have spent vast swaths of time these last few days sitting in one of those standard-issue IKEA chairs with a bent wood frame that runs along the floor, curves up for legs, then bends horizontally again for arms, and connected to a frame that arcs upward for the back. It bends back a bit under pressure and has a matching footstool. Due to the curvature, it even rocks gently. I have a premium model with leather cushions that I bought from a neighbour when she was moving. I sit in front of a big patio window that magnifies the sunshine and ... well ... just relax. I tell myself, not falsely I think, that this is what recovery looks like.

Sometimes I read or listen to music, but often not. When not, I'm known to drift in and out of a gentle sleep. Spending so much time doing next to nothing isn't an activity (if you can call it that) that I thought I would ever enjoy, at least not for another 30 years. I certainly hope that it's not corrupting ...

Rex, the dog, and I also take walks in the woods. Sometimes my wife or son comes along. My only risk of excessive ambition these days is when taking these walks. There is an old Jewish cemetery about 5 km through the woods from our place. They stopped interning the bodies of the departed there at the end of the nineteenth century. Being a couple of hundred years old, it feels ancient to an American. It lies at the edge of the woods and fields of fruit trees. I sometimes walk there and add a stone of remembrance to a collection on the roughhewn stone pillars at the gate. We have had a steady succession of glorious early spring days, which have encouraged me to walk. Rex and I set out for the graveyard on Saturday. He enjoys it because leash laws don't apply to the last stretch and to the area outside the cemetery. Our walk there was sunny and delightful. But on the way back, I began to feel the exhaustion, my pace slowed considerably, and I looked for benches to rest on. I wondered if I would have to send him home like Lassie, with a message that I needed rescue. In time, we did make it home, and I was chastened to think of every walk in terms of the round trip involved.

My appetite still suffers a bit, and I am distressed that the food that I love does not taste as it should. I suppose lots of taste buds were collateral damage from the chemotherapy. My eyelashes were as well. My eyelids itch and the corners of my eyes burn. I have my first post-release follow-up doctor's appointment tomorrow, and I am hoping that my doctor can provide me with some kind of relief for the eyes.

35
A Thread of Good Fortune

Today, I had my second follow-up appointment with my doctor after leaving the hospital. He was happy with how things were going. The blood counts continue to improve and the side effects, limited so far mainly to fatigue, and the occasional nausea and diarrhoea, are typical.

I learned a few things. For example, the transplant nurse explained to me that the sources of fatigue are not particularly well understood, but that I could expect it to vary from day to day and that it could last six months, possibly even a year. I also learned that the fibrosis that was scarring my bone marrow and inhibiting blood production does not simply disappear when the old bone marrow is killed and the new develops. Rather, it disappears only slowly over time, and probably never fully. But it will be very significantly diminished and will not degenerate further. So, it will not pose any health threats.

The continued presence of the fibrosis explains why, when they performed another bone marrow biopsy today - my fourth in a year, but hey who's counting? - they had such difficulty finding blood in my marrow. It was the familiar process of anaesthetizing the muscle tissue outside the hip bone, and then with great force puncturing the bone, causing a sharp pain from deep within that made me want to squeal, and finally turning the big firm needle this way and that way to extract a core of the marrow for laboratory study. The problem was that they didn't only want marrow, they also wanted a sample of blood from inside the marrow. Sadly, that was not to be found on the first *four* attempts at ramming the large needle into my hip. So, they made one last courageous attempt and, in the end, came up with a very small sample, which they hoped would be enough. I hoped so too.

Apparently, I will have to endure this a couple more times in the next year, as they study the retreat of the fibrosis.

This afternoon I succumbed to the fatigue and rested on the couch. But I found myself strangely bothered. I couldn't help but think about how contingent my good fortune and the success of the transplant up to this point had been, how much harder it might have been, and how it might not have worked at all. A thread of fortune had supported me, kept me from falling into dire circumstances. Some day that thread breaks for all of us. I couldn't chase away these thoughts and was sufficiently exercised by them that I didn't really sleep or even rest all that much. So it goes. Those were, I think, episodic thoughts. Fortunately, nothing like that has been able to fight back against the exhaustion at night. And I don't expect tonight to be different.

36 Magical Thinking

I don't know what it's like to get a stage four cancer diagnosis. I wouldn't want to pretend to speak with authority about what an emotional punch in the solar plexus that must be. Still, I get angry when I read stories on the internet of people having cured themselves of metastatic cancer by doing nothing more than drinking carrot juice. The same goes for people claiming that our thoughts can cause and cure cancer I have no truck with consuming carrots, positive thinking, or prayer. My objection is to the medical claims, the causal efficacy, if you will, of these activities for curing illness.

I do know a little about having a life-threatening illness; and I know something about the anxiety a diagnosis can produce. And I can imagine why some people would prefer almost anything to chemotherapy, especially if they have already experienced how crappy it makes them feel. I can conceive of why someone might seek alternatives to conventional medical care, especially if their prognosis is poor. Still, I think that the pursuit of these alternatives is a big mistake and that to encourage people to engage in them is irresponsible.

To rely on *alternatives* to conventional medicine, such as drinking carrot juice or thinking positively is to trust one's life to magical thinking. The fundamental feature of magical thinking is the rejection of the scientific picture of how the world works. This is a picture that includes the idea that biological conditions, such as wellness and illness in organisms, are caused by other biological processes and other physical influences, such as trauma. And that medical science can, in many instances, affect these biological processes and improve the condition of patients.

The scientific picture of the world posits a causal relationship between a biological condition, such as illness, and some possible influence on the existence of repeated experimentation. Medical science is exceedingly complex, and much is not very well understood. So, it's possible that what looks like a relation of causation is instead some sort of statistical fluke. We can't be certain without being able to repeat the sequence of apparent cause and effect, preferably on a large scale. Evidence-based medicine is supported through such processes of repetition and large-scale study.

Magical thinking involves affirming and disseminating views that are not supported by the evidence in that way and that generally do not seem to fit very well with our current evidence of the way the world works. This makes the claims of magical thinking highly suspect.

Magical thinking can lead to false hope. It can encourage patients to put their aspirations and emotional resources in the service of an effort that is doomed to fail. Moreover, too often, magical thinking involves claims about the control that individuals have over their wellness that are implicitly victim blaming.

Our world is through and through full of the results of scientific enquiry and experiment applied to the development of infrastructure, technology, medicines, and medical procedures. Most of us don't think much about the physics involved in the engineering of bridges as we drive over them. We simply trust that the bridge will hold us. The contrary happens so rarely that it is perfectly sensible not to worry about it. We fundamentally trust in the sciences and engineering to live the way we do. Just think of how much more difficult our lives would be, the prospects for surgery, for example, without the discovery of Penicillin and the subsequent development of antibiotics.

The trust we have in science and engineering should give us reason to pause when we are encouraged to forgo it by the offer of a cure that is at odds with the conventional scientific understanding of how causes work in the physical world. And magical thinking is precisely that.

Our basic trust in science is one reason to believe that magical thinking offers false hope. Another is based on economics. Think about how much cheaper it would be to treat cancer by means of carrots than chemotherapy. Prayer would be cheaper still. If these worked reliably as alternatives, insurers - whether private or public - would have a very strong incentive to nudge, even shove, us all in that direction. It would be a terrible waste of their money for us to receive chemotherapy. As we all know, private insurers make it their business to figure out ways to cut the costs of the services they cover in order to boost their profits. Unless you think insurers are not particularly cost conscious, the fact that they do not push us to consume carrots or to pray instead of taking chemotherapy should give you a compelling reason to doubt that either carrot juice and prayer can serve as alternatives for curing cancer.

It is much more likely that a patient will find a cure, manage their symptoms, or gain palliative relief if they trust in the accumulated understanding of medical science. Such understanding is imperfect to be sure, and it will not always be able to deliver what patients want most dearly, but there is no more reliable alternative towards better health.

If magical thinking only encouraged false hope, it would be bad enough. But it is sometimes even worse still. At least some forms of magical thinking claim that a more positive or prayerful outlook on the world can reliably prevent serious disease and cure it when it occurs. If that were the case, then those who were gravely ill would have it within their control to cure themselves. By implication, if they remain sick, then the failure is theirs. This is victim blaming pure and simple. To friends and relatives of patients, any suggestion of this to a terribly ill person would be deeply offensive.

37 Hope Kept Me Eating

The ancient Greek poet Hesiod recounts a tale of the origin of suffering. Pandora opened a jar stuffed full of evils by the Olympian gods. As a result, 'countless plagues, wander amongst men; for earth is full of evils, and the sea is full ... diseases come upon men continually by day and by night, bringing mischief to mortals' (Hesiod 1914: Lines 100–05). But curiously, that jar was closed before hope was also allowed to escape.

What are we to make of that? The moral of the legend is ambiguous. Is it an expression of how bleak the human condition is? There really is no hope. But if we could somehow reopen the jar, at least we would have some hope. Or is the idea instead that hope is also an evil, like disease, and accessing it will bring us even further torment, the torment of disappointment? The nineteenth-century philosopher Nietzsche took a version of the latter interpretation. Hope is among the greatest of evils because it prolongs our torment (Nietzsche 1996: I. 71). Acceptance is far better than hope. Let us not imagine something better, but say 'yes' to the world as it is. That's a view that seems curiously close to a kind of Stoicism. Better to focus on the here and now, that which we might control, than to project into the future, which is far beyond our control.

In my diagnosis of magical thinking, I worried that in desperation patients often embrace false hopes. We often fix on alternatives to conventional medicine and, in doing so, forego the more reliable path to a cure, to a longer life, or to palliative relief. When we do that, it seems as if hope is not our friend. In those instances, hope becomes a servant of disease.

So, it does seem that there can be a danger in hoping. Even the great philosopher of hope, Ernst Bloch, claimed that 'there is no hope without anxiety' (1995: 333). As a Stoic might claim, when we project ourselves into the future, we open ourselves up to anxiety just as much as to hope. If we are concerned about preventing anxiety, maybe it would be better to redirect our attention to the present and foreclose both anxiety and hope. Make no mistake about it; Nietzsche's counsel is not one of despair. On the contrary, he believes that we can only fully affirm the present by foregoing hope.

But I ask you, could anyone ever really do that? Could a patient so fully live in the present as to have neither anxiety nor hope? Bloch, at least, was doubtful. He asserted that forward-looking projection is fundamental to the kind of minds we have. Like a lighthouse, we are constantly seeking to illuminate our future, and in fact it is only because of that that progress is possible (Bloch 1995: 295–97).

If there are situations in which hope seems counterproductive, just try to imagine a world completely without hope. All criticism of the present would be left without a strategic goal, and it could easily fall victim to cynicism. Imagine if the abolitionists had no hope. Martin Luther King, Jr. was fond of quoting the abolitionist Rev. Theodore Parker, who during the height of the transatlantic slave trade dared to say: 'I do not pretend to understand the moral universe; I cannot calculate the curve and complete the figure by experience of sight; I can divine it by conscience. And from what I see I am sure it bends towards justice' (1853: 84–85). Could Martin Luther King Jr. have been the strategic leader of the civil rights movement without hope? Could Nelson Mandela have led the African National Congress from a prison cell on Robbin Island without hope? Hope is a powerful aid to action. It can play a service role by impelling us to act when our motivation may be weakening.

At two different points while I was in the hospital, hope kept me eating. One of the side effects of the kind of chemotherapy that was administered to me was to shutdown of the production of saliva in my mouth as well as the mucus throughout my digestive tract. My mouth was as dry as the great Mojave Desert. Eating became a chore. I would be given a roll at breakfast, and when I took a bite and began chewing, I might as well have been sucking on sand. I was miserable and had nothing but aversion to food. The only thing keeping me going was the hope of getting stronger. If I were to weaken myself by insufficient intake of calories, I would delay my recovery. And so, I ate.

Later, I contracted a gastrointestinal infection, and I was plagued by severe diarrhoea. I was losing weight. My appetite was also on the wane because the chemotherapy had inflicted heavy damage on my taste buds. Most foods did not taste good (many still don't) and some were positively revolting. The nurses would occasionally warn that if I were to lose much more weight, I would have to be put on a nutritional IV at night. I had to eat much more at each meal than I felt comfortable. It was unpleasant, both because there was so much food and because none of it tasted very good. The hope of renewed strength kept me eating.

There is another thing that the political struggles I mentioned demonstrate. We don't typically hope alone. A community of hope supports people hoping. The leaders are buoyed by the inspiring sacrifices of the members of the struggle, and the members are carried along by the fierce commitment and rhetorical elegance of the leaders. And my efforts of personal hope were supported by the love of family and friends, near and far, many of whom offered inspiring comments across the ocean via the internet.

Hope is an aid in tough times. When it's well-placed, hope can help us in the effort to transform our circumstances, in the effort to fix what needs mending. From illness in our bodies to the injustices in our institutions, there is no shortage of things needing fixing. But in motivating us to change our condition, hope can also change us. Hope plays not only a service role in helping us to achieve our ends. Hope can transform us by increasing our agency. Sometimes, as in the case of the abolitionist movement, the civil rights movement, and the anti-apartheid movement, we are acting to secure human dignity. By enhancing our capacity to be agents of dignity, hope gives expression to our own dignity. Hope can have a dignity-expressing function.

I am not claiming that I left the hospital a more dignified person. The kind of dignity that I am talking about is not measured along a scale like weight or wealth. It is possessed equally by everyone. And although hope allowed me to express a certain determination to be healthy again, it was my own survival at stake, not the protection of the dignity of others. In hope, I was no hero. Hope in the hospital is different in that way from hope in the streets. Nonetheless, in both cases, hope gives expression to something that we admire in people. And our lives would be far poorer if we had to live without it.

38 Sunshine, Suffering, Rebirth, and Freedom

I'm sitting in the standard-issue IKEA chair, and I'm wearing an industrial-strength white face mask because I have the sliding doors wide open, exposing me to airborne micro-nasties. These things have a revolting polymer stench to them. The sun is warming me while the fresh breeze is cooling me. Rex is alongside me, allowing the sun's rays to warm his black body. The patients back in the transplant unit are stuck in their stuffy rooms with only their imaginations to torture them over the pleasures they are missing on this delightful Good Friday morning. We patients pass through those rooms in trickles, and with good luck, time in the sunshine will soon come to the patients now in the transplant unit. I imagine them humming the Animals' classic anthem, 'We Gotta Get Out of This Place'.

Kant argues that we would be people of better, more sensitive moral dispositions if we were to visit the sick in the hospitals and asylums (1996: 205 6:457). Given his moral rationalism, that comment confounds some readers. But regardless of the ultimate basis of morality, a vivid understanding of how we can suffer in body and mind can surely aid us in understanding how we can help others. And according to Kant, one of the two great principles of moral life is love; the other is justice (1996: 230 6:488).

Due to the enforced isolation, when you are a patient in the transplant unit, you don't see much of the suffering of others. But, of course, you are bound to go through some yourself. I do remember clearly, on my last day, when I shared a room for a few hours with two other men, one came in deeply dejected, having returned to the unit after several months of good health on the outside. He had developed diarrhoea, and the doctors needed to determine whether he was suffering from some kind of graft vs. host disease. That's when the new donor immune system begins to attack the organs of one's body as if they are threatening outsiders. It's a bit like adopting a Pit Bull to protect you, but because it perceives you, not the bad guys, as the threat, it goes after you. He sat in his bed, his head bent, and his spirit seemed broken. His elderly parents looked helplessly on. That memory serves as a reminder that so often, physical suffering is accompanied by deep mental anguish. As Kant seems to recommend, witnessing that might remind us of our common human frailty. We could use more such reminders these days. In public discussions, refugees are often presented as threats to our collective security rather than people who are deeply traumatized and profoundly suffering.

Lent is nearly over, and it is about the midpoint of Passover. I had hoped to be free of the disease and in possession of a new immune system by the end of Lent, and by great good fortune that is the case. But for the next six months or so, a disappointing return to the hospital due to complications of one kind or another is not out of the question. I have the immune system of a newborn, and I need to be as careful as one is with a newborn when it comes to exposure to germs. One consequence of this is that over the next few months, I will need once again to receive all of the childhood vaccinations - mumps, measles, etc. (And I think you can imagine what I might think of the views of the anti-vaccination crowd.) Meanwhile, I hope that the new Pit Bull-like force in my body knows who its master is.

But with each passing day, it's a bit less likely that serious problems will arise. I passed a milestone this week. Yesterday, my doctor told me that

I could reduce my check-up visits to once a week, rather than twice. And blood tests reveal that 99–100 percent of the blood in my body now originates from the new stem cells. The transplant has been, at least initially, a resounding success.

39
Food Aversions

I've been thinking. They should warn patients before chemotherapy that there is a risk that whatever they eat during or around that time will be utterly repellent to them later. But here's the problem. Once eating becomes a chore, you seek out old standbys for comfort and satisfaction. Nonetheless, the very idea of potato chips right now is almost enough to make me wretch. Sparkling water is out of the question. Spaghetti, especially al dente as the pizza place near the hospital made it, is borderline. Fortunately, yogurt still holds its appeal. But I may never eat boiled potatoes again. No great loss there.

I suppose this too will pass.

I am grateful that, in their great wisdom, the good doctors did not allow me to drink beer and red wine in the hospital.

40 Inching Towards Normalcy

The doctor's visit yesterday brought more good news. He further reduced the medications. I'm now only taking about 15 pills a day! That's about half of what I was taking when I was first discharged, nearly four weeks ago now. The main noticeable effects of the reduced medicine intake are that I am bothered far less often by the occasional nausea and diarrhoea. Certainly welcome effects!

He also relaxed some of the rules around the house. I am allowed to bathe now. That's in addition to showering, perhaps I should add! I can handle the dirty dishes and take out the trash. My house partners will waste no time putting me to work.

I still have to avoid groups of people, however, which means I won't be attending the upcoming Bob Dylan concert. I know, I know, he is often not in top form live. Still, I would have gone. I saw him one time in Hollywood when he was really on. It keeps you hoping.

While working out today, I felt stronger than at any time since entering the hospital. And I could visualize feeling normal again. For the first 18 of the last 19 years, the thought that my chronic disease might morph into a life-threatening disease was never buried very deep. I rarely dwelled on it. But I could call it to mind easily enough. Then, from last spring onwards, as the planning for the transplant was just beginning, I would wonder to myself where, or if, I would be in a year. I remember telling my wife how strange it seemed, how open the future seemed. You make plans, of course. But you also make contingency plans. I planned my memorial service, for example. During the lead-up to the transplant, the possibility of failure loomed ever present on the horizon of my thinking. That's all gone now. And I can imagine full health being just around the corner. That's also strange in its own way after so long. But wonderfully so.

41 Human Fatigue and Canine Anxiety

I have the feeling that I'll have more energy today. The energy business is difficult. When I lack it, when fatigue really falls like a leaden blanket, I'm left defenceless. The standard-issue IKEA chair beckons to me. And I'm reduced to nodding off while doing nothing in particular. It affects everything about my experience of the day. It's the difference between just sitting limply in the chair and responding enthusiastically to emails, between dragging myself up the stairs and ascending with gusto, between reading with engaged interest and succumbing to sleep before I know whether Levin will go meet Kitty at her sister's country residence. Fatigue is not some additional thing to deal with in the day; it's the way the whole day is experienced.

I'm glad that I was warned about it. Otherwise, I'd have been seriously worried when the blanket of lethargy fell unannounced. When it smothers you, there's nothing to be done really, but to check out, put all plans on hold, and hope that no one is disappointed and no deadlines are blown.

I had a long string of good days last week. So good that I began to think that I was now beyond concerns about fatigue. But I learned as a child that, 'Pride goeth before destruction, and an haughty spirit before a fall' (Proverbs 16:18 1987). Sunday arrived and I was confined to the IKEA chair. Ugh. I rebounded enough on Monday to get some work done and to exercise.

Tuesday began well enough. I attended my first-ever hospital yoga class, which in itself was an exercise in humility. It was also socially interesting. There were only four of us in the class, and two of us were still bald. Although we were all four from different countries, we were also all veterans of the haematology/oncology department. We shared a comradery, like soldiers who had been in the same battle.

The appointment at the clinic dragged on as the doctor expressed concern that my creatinine level at 2.1 was way too high. I run chronically high in this regard in any case, but clearly my kidneys were being stressed by a combination of some medication and my failure to drink enough. He ordered a change of medication and sent me off to the day clinic to receive a hydration IV. The whole experience at the hospital lasted about seven hours. Alas, another day offered in sacrifice for longevity. It left me chastened. I need to keep track of my fluid intake, just like the nagging nurses required of me in the transplant unit. At home, I had quickly shrugged off their imposed discipline - I prefer my discipline self-imposed - for a more 'intuitive' approach. Surprise, surprise, that seems not to be working.

At my request, on my way back home, the taxi driver dropped me off at the pharmacy. From there, I walked about a kilometre home. As I approached our house, it was clear that Rex was having a bad day, too. I could hear him howling from the road along which our row of houses sits. Anxiety had set in at some point, and I wondered how long he'd been in such a panic. How do dogs experience anxiety? Is he imagining some future all alone, the pack never returning? That seems unlikely. Epictetus's diagnosis that anxiety is caused by allowing images of an uncertain future to worry us seems to require more powers of projection than I suspect dogs possess. Is it just the absence of companions in the present that becomes intolerable? Maybe after a while, the voice of the BBC broadcaster, which I leave on for him, fails to soothe. But why, then, does it only happen after some period of time passes? Given our common mammalian heritage, interpreting the behaviour as anxiety analogous to what humans experience seems right. But how analogous?

By the time I got settled at home, I had about an hour's worth of energy to work on a manuscript before the crushing weight of fatigue sent me to the chair. Fortunately, my wife had already volunteered to cook dinner and with *almost* no grumbling my son was convinced to walk Rex. So, I had the rest of the time before dinner and all of it afterwards to consider the contours of the chair before hauling myself upstairs to bed. After ten or so hours of sleep, I feel well-rested today.

One consequence of the new medication regimen is that I am back to a twice-a-week schedule of visiting the doctor for the next couple of weeks. I've laid off a certain anti-viral pill in favour of an antiprotozoal substance that is ingested by means of a vaporizer. It is administered at the hospital on a weekly basis. So, I go back to the doctor again on Friday to breathe it all in. I'm sorry that Rex will be home alone. I hope to make it back before the anxiety starts up. There's no convincing him that I will be back before too long.

42
Healthcare for All Pt. 3

The hospital bill finally arrived in the mail today. It is for €280 for 28 days of care in isolation and a life-saving stem cell transplant. Mandatory payroll tax-financed health insurance is just so tyrannical. When will the masses revolt against it?

43
Still Wearing My Helmet

I took Rex for a walk this evening. As I was enjoying the golden light of the sunset filtering through the green foliage of the woods and the birdsong all around me, I realized that two days ago was the one-year anniversary of my diagnosis. A year ago, after I left the office of the squat doctor, I met my wife in the evening at a reception at a humanities research centre near our house. She had ridden her bike to the centre after teaching all day, and I rode over from our house. As we were heading out to our bikes after the reception, I mentioned to her that I needed to talk to her about my appointment that day. She knew that I was going to receive my biopsy results. She looked at me seriously, but then joked, 'So are you going to start riding without a helmet?' Her way of asking if the prognosis is bad. I replied, 'Well no ... not yet ... but I think I need to do some more research.' Then I explained that the biopsy was positive for *myelofibrosis*. Neither of us was exactly sure what that meant, but she could tell that it wasn't good news.

A year ago, we had no idea what was in store for us the coming year. I never went back for another appointment with that doctor. Instead, I sought a second opinion, switched doctors, and never looked back. I now realize that, given the diagnosis, things could not have gone more smoothly this past year. But it has been an exercise in coming to terms with the reality that the orientation of one's life can switch dramatically from one day to the next, and not always for the better. And that possibility - let's face it - is always there for all of us. As the Preacher in Ecclesiastes observes:

> [T]he race is not to the swift, nor the battle to the strong, neither yet bread to the wise, nor yet riches to men of understanding, nor yet favour to men of skill; but time and chance happeneth to them all. For man also knoweth not his time: as the fishes that are taken in an evil net, and as the birds that are caught in the snare; so are the sons of men snared in an evil time, when it falleth suddenly upon them.
>
> (9:11-12)

The message of Ecclesiastes is not supposed to be one of despair. At one point, the Preacher also recommends, 'Go thy way, eat thy bread with joy, and drink thy wine with a merry heart' (Ecclesiastes 9:7). The contingency of life and the inevitability of hard times are no reason for nihilism. All that is valuable does not lose its value simply because life is temporary and highly contingent. To think otherwise seems remarkably solipsistic. The finitude of life provides a reason to make the most of the time that we have to learn, love, grow, create, and improve the world around us. Not to give up on all that.

With the transplant behind me and the recovery moving along nicely, the orientation of our own lives is slowly shifting again, and most certainly for the better. I hope to be wearing my helmet for many years to come.

44
Same as It Ever Was

I continue to let the days go by. That's been harder than it sounds. Not that I have any big complaints about my physical condition. I really couldn't have asked for things to go any better. If you have to go through this, I don't imagine it could be much easier than I've had it so far. I've been out of the hospital for nearly two months now, and I have not had a single incidence of fever, vomiting, or prolonged diarrhoea - the kinds of things that send you back to the emergency room. I still suffer from food aversions and a weak appetite. I've lost about ten pounds, but nobody seems worried about that. I am not particularly weak although I am weaker, of course, than when I went into the hospital. Still, the last three weeks I've managed to work out - cardio and weights - three days a week and go to yoga once a week. Ice cream and pie have kept the calories coming in. Lately, I have been specializing in baking fresh blueberry pies. They are a crowd pleaser.

In January, about six weeks before the transplant, I injured my left knee running. X-rays revealed nothing. I did not have time to get an MRI before the transplant, but the pain persisted. I had to give up running and switched to a spin bike at home and then a stationary bike in the hospital. When I first got out of the hospital, Rex and I went for walks in the woods and I used the spin bike again, but this past week the knee felt good enough for a couple of short and slow runs in the woods. Running in the fresh air lifted the spirits of both the canine and the human.

No, I have no reason to complain about my physical condition. I know people who have had it much rougher afterwards. People for whom the new immune system decided that the old bodily organs were a threat. Graft vs. host disease can be a serious problem. The graft, the new immune system, can go after any organ in the body, the host that it registers as foreign. That's why I am on immune suppressants, which increase my risk of infection. When you talk about this, you'll notice, it's really hard not to ascribe agency and intelligence to the immune system: it 'decides'; it 'goes after', it 'registers'. All of this, as if the immune system is a homunculus perceiving its environment and deciding to act according to its purposes. This is really no explanation at all, since you're left explaining how a bodily system works by positing some little dwarf inside acting, but then there must be an even smaller dwarf in him, and so on. Although it seems so natural to ascribe intelligence and agency to systems within us, in fact it obscures a difficult and fascinating problem. How does this all work anyway? What is the causal explanation for why the immune system might 'recognize' an organ as a threat and 'direct' an attack against it? And how can it be explained without an infinite army of ever smaller homunculi?

I remember talking to my haematologist before the transplant about blood production. She was explaining that as the bone marrow becomes more scarred and produces less blood, the spleen and liver slowly, but increasingly, take over more and more of the blood production. That is surprising enough since it's not their function to produce blood, but somehow, they have the capacity to do so. But I found another question even more fascinating: how do they 'know' to start to produce blood and then to produce more? She smiled and said, 'That's still a mystery.' That doctors can carry off a stem cell transplant and save a person's life is evidence that medical science understands a lot, but that they don't know what causes the liver and spleen to begin producing blood and how that cause is related to the bone marrow producing less blood shows how much more there is to learn. It's crazy.

Anyway, I am physically well, considering it all. I was warned that my recovery would take at least six months, and possibly as long as twelve months. Still, I am frustrated and impatient. I am well enough to feel pretty damn good much of the time although I still proceed more ploddingly than normal, and my wife assures me that I am sometimes a bit confused - although I can't say that I have noticed it!

My situation reminds me of those little dogs I see in the woods that are on very long retractable leads. The leashes are so long that they run along, tail wagging, thinking they are free. That is until the owner pulls the trigger and the lead pulls them back in. Every once in a while, after I have been running along with my tail wagging, I get yanked back and find myself plopped in the IKEA chair or lying on the couch with little will or energy to do much of anything else the entire day.

It's in a kind of purgatory. There is every reason to be hopeful that I will just continue to get better. Slowly. But in the meantime, despite often feeling good, I move more slowly, accomplish things less quickly, spend my life mostly in the house, and I must reckon with unannounced and unwelcome fatigue. It's been that way for several weeks now and will probably remain so for some time still to come.

45 Who Is That Masked Man?

By the doctor's orders, I wear a surgical face mask outside of the house. It's green, three-ply, and has elastic bands that wrap around my ears. It has an accordion-style construction that allows expansion so as to pull it down below my chin and up above my nostrils. It sits on the bridge of my nose, and near its top edge, it has a piece of wire that bends to fit snugly on the bridge of the nose and down the sides onto the cheekbone. The wire serves to close the gap there. But despite that, exhalation still escapes at the top and often fogs my glasses, which are not equipped with a defrost system. That's just one of the annoyances of wearing the mask. This kind of mask is a more comfortable step down from what I used to wear. It was a thicker, form-fitted white thing with a built-in filter near the front. The smell from the inside was repulsive.

Apart from walks with Rex in the woods, my getting out has been limited, again by doctor's orders, to going to the clinic for check-ups and getting meds from the pharmacy. I wear the mask in the taxi - funded by public health insurance - to and from the doctor and to the pharmacy. My driver is used to me carrying on my side of our conversation through the mask. He is Afghan and has a son a year younger than mine. Our weekly topics range from children and schools to the Taliban and ISIS. The few times I have been in town, people have mostly politely ignored the existence of the mask. Children often stare, but adults in this culture mostly do not smile at strangers on the streets anyway and seem trained just to look past. In the pharmacy, of course, the employees are professional. They are as indifferent to me as they would be to any other customer.

I'm a foreigner. This might not be obvious to locals by appearance, but as soon as I begin to speak it is. My accent marks me as 'other' right away. Typically, the locals are very gracious about my German ability. I've made an effort to learn the language, and I can have a conversation respectably. I get nothing but praise and encouragement for my efforts. Being a foreigner, however, means that I am not always sure how to respond to people. Sometimes I seek confirmation from local friends to understand responses from people that seem off to me; I've been assured, for example, that another neighbour two houses down in our row really is the one being outrageous and not me when she yells in response to my firing up the gas grill.

Who Is That Masked Man?

The face mask has presented me with new interpretive problems. I mentioned that people don't tend in any case to be warm with strangers, unless you are with a dog. Perfect stranger to his human companion. Twice in the last two months while walking in the woods, Rex and I have been approached by strangers, asking after no more than a cursory greeting if I were wearing the mask because I am especially sensitive to something in the woods. Both times, I was taken aback. To me, the familiarity seemed odd, almost rude, especially in a country where passersby routinely ignore one another. In both cases, however, I spontaneously put together an elevator speech version of my recent health history.

Afterwards, as self-entertainment, I've wondered what else I could have said? A few thoughts have crossed my mind. Perhaps, 'Oh the mask, that's just so that I don't infect you with my deadly disease.' Period. Silence. Or maybe, 'No, I'm not from around here, and I'm just not sure how sanitary you all are.' But, of course, the idea that I should take offense at the strangers' questions just might be a cultural miscue on my part, like firing up the gas grill.

46 Inspiration in the Oncology/ Haematology Waiting Room

If they had their druthers, nobody would be waiting in this particular room, the one everyone hopes never to have to visit. The dreaded room, the room of the cursed. Like a soldier sitting in a room waiting to be shipped off to war, looking around and wondering who will return alive, you can find yourself wondering about the other patients, their stage, and their prognoses. Boredom mixed with morbid curiosity and empathy leads to such speculation. Some people chat as if they are continuing conversations they started somewhere else, perhaps from many appointments on the same day or from spending time together in the chemotherapy room.

But mostly, people don't talk while they wait. One time, I had a guy sitting next to me who seemed to be barely conscious. Before long, he started to spray blood out of the top of his hand where a bandage had just fallen off. I leaned away, and his wife yelled in panic. The nurses came running, whisked him away, and cleaned up the mess. That's far more excitement than anyone wants in that room, and thankfully, far more than we usually get. Typically, we wait in silence, alone with our worries, our hopes, and our morbid curiosities.

There is a fairly long wait between the drawing of the blood and the consultation with a doctor, where the blood counts are discussed. In between, the blood has to be sent to the lab and analysed, and the results must be entered into the computer system. The waiting time varies between 30 minutes and two hours. So, this past week I decided to get a cup of coffee after my blood was drawn. When I returned to the waiting room, I found an open seat, adjacent to which were the belongings of someone who must have been in the back room having blood drawn. I couldn't remember who might be sitting there, but since people tend not to socialize, I didn't much care. I'm nearly done with *Anna Karenina*, and I was looking forward to diving into the book. I plopped down and got busy with the book. A few minutes later, a woman five to ten years my elder sat down. Apparently, she looked over to see what I was reading because she immediately said something to the effect of how nice it was that I was reading *that* book. I wasn't looking for conversation, and I certainly didn't expect it, but I was about to get it.

I didn't really want to stop reading, so I replied pleasantly but briefly and returned to the book. But she would not relent. I soon learned that she was from Brazil. After meeting the man who would be her husband on a Pacific cruise about ten years ago, they each returned home to their respective countries. But then he contacted her telling her that he had a cancerous growth on his throat. She decided to move halfway across the world to help with his care. She left behind a grown daughter and elderly mother. At some point after that, they were married. But he's been in and out of the hospital ever since. The details of it all were a bit hard to follow because I was having some trouble with her thick Portuguese accent. So, we switched to English, a language we were both more comfortable in. She told me that while he was in the hospital, initially she kept herself busy by learning guitar and singing, first in a Protestant choir and then in a Catholic one. I didn't ask if she switched for musical or theological reasons. A few years back, her own health troubles began. Her platelet counts dropped precipitously for unknown reasons. In response, she was treated with a high dose of cortisone, which elicited psychotic reactions. The doctors switched to chemotherapy and that seems to be helping. And although she has no one to help her out, she has also been taking care of her husband all along.

She related this whole story without a complaint, an indication of regret, or a trace of self-pity. It was just her life that she was telling me about. I marvelled at her strength and spirit. The discussion lasted for at least half an hour, but she was eventually called into the back room for her doctor's consultation. When she came out, before leaving, she came over to me, smiled, shook my hand, and pleasantly said goodbye. The Stoic philosopher Marcus Aurelius advised that we should strive to be like the cliff against which the waves continually crash, but standing firm tames the fury of the waves; for then we will not be unhappy due to what has happened to us, but remain happy despite what happens (2017: 57). We don't know how we are going to react to hardship when it falls on us, but I could only hope to have her fortitude and sanguinity. I never learned her name, but I may never forget our remarkable conversation.

47
With a Little Help from My Friends

I've been preoccupied with two pictures of personhood since the last post about my encounter with the woman in the waiting room. One is Aurelius's cliff, standing firm against the crashing sea. The strength of the rock to stand up against the relentless pounding forces of nature, the decay and destruction of aging and illness, offers an example of a way to live that is meant to secure happiness in the face of calamity. Nature, of course, ultimately wins. Eventually, the sea will cause the cliff to erode and crash into the turbulent waters, just as certainly as illness and death come to us all, but the idea is that happiness consists in standing strong for as long as one can. The Stoics generally argue that we do so by relinquishing what in any case cannot be kept, and ultimately this includes our lives. Doing so, they know, is no easy feat.

Epictetus begins his manual on stoic philosophy, *The Enchiridion*, by noting that, 'there are things which are within our power, and there are things which are beyond our power' (1983: 1). It is important to remind ourselves in which category each of the things we hold dear belongs, so that we do not allow ourselves to make our happiness dependent on what we cannot control. This extends to family and friends. 'If you wish your children and your wife and your friends to live forever, you are foolish, for you wish things to be in your power that are not so' (Epictetus 1983: 14). The aim to be able to let go of all that one holds dear might sound familiar to Buddhists (Mirodha Bodhi 2000: 56.11). 'Never say of anything, "I have lost it", but "I have restored it". Has your child died? It is restored. Has your wife died? She is restored' (Epictetus 1983: 11). By letting go of it all, the Stoic philosopher can then accept all that happens to her, in the end even death. 'Demand not that events should be as you wish; but wish them to happen as they do happen, and you will go on well' (Epictetus 1983: 8). As I mentioned earlier, this is a life without hope; hope is only needed by those who would have events go as they wish. That is precisely what is to be avoided.

The Stoic ideal of strength is in many ways admirable. But can one be happy with such an attitude towards those whom one loves most? Or does a full, rich, and happy life require making oneself vulnerable to the loss of all that enriches one's life and the people whom one loves? Just as I have already cast doubt on the ability and desirability of living without hope, which the Stoics seem to recommend, so I also find doubtful the Stoic picture of a person so radically alone.

The second picture comes from John Donne. Perhaps he had Aurelius's cliff image in mind when he penned these words: 'If a clod be washed away to sea Europe is the less' (Donne 1999: 45). When Donne wrote this, he may have been embracing a Pauline notion of the Body of Christ, but the image of solidarity expressed in these and other words of *Meditation XVII* are also available to those who interpret life through a purely secular lens. When, in the nineteenth century, John Stuart Mill sought to provide an account of a progressive morality entirely on secular grounds of human happiness, he also had an inspiring vision of what human solidarity could do:

> All the grand sources, in short, of human suffering are in great degree, many of them almost entirely, conquerable by human care and effort [...]. [E]very mind sufficiently intelligent and generous to bear a part, however small and unconspicuous, in the endeavour, will draw a noble enjoyment from the contest itself, which he would not for any bribe in the form of selfish indulgence consent to be without.
>
> (2004: 34)

We all rely crucially upon others to become who we are and to thrive in the activities of making a life. From the cradle to the hospice room, we make our lives together, even if we fancy we live all alone on a libertarian archipelago. As I have mentioned before, I owe my life to an anonymous donor and a social-democratic healthcare system. Mine and my family's well-being is owed to all the friends who helped and supported us while I was in the hospital. The community that I enjoyed through the comments to this blog helped me to fight off anxiety and loneliness while I was otherwise isolated in the hospital.

The Stoics have important lessons to teach us about finding happiness in letting go of much that we cannot control, including coming to accept the inevitability of our own deaths. But I doubt that the Stoic sense of individualism can give the social character of our well-being its due. Can we be in love, in friendship, and in solidarity with others whom we can simply let be 'restored'? I think not, and Epictetus might agree. In fact, that may be the point. The commitments of love and solidarity necessarily render us vulnerable to the losses experienced by others and to our loss when we lose them. But these commitments also literally give us life and enrich it. Invulnerability is neither a possibility nor an ideal worthy of our striving. One might suspect that there may be something tragic in that state of affairs. But given what's to be lived, it's not so clear that, on balance, it's tragic, rather than just human.

48 Springtime on My Face

It may be summer outside now, but it's still springtime on my face and head. Like crocuses peeking out from the ground in April, early this month, the hair under my nose started to bust through my skin. After a while, I had a passable moustache and a scraggly goatee. My scalp, in comparison, has been lagging. At first, some adolescent peach fuzz appeared up there. I shaved this stuff twice. I told myself that doing so was necessary, like on a pubescent boy's cheeks, to get the real manly stuff to grow (where it still would) on top. But the truth is that I have gotten used to the bald scalp, recently supplemented by a moustache and goatee. I am told variously that I look like Mr. Clean, Michel Foucault, and Telly Savalas. (Bruce Willis has not come up.) I flatter myself that these are meant as compliments. But after going bowling for my wife's birthday, a friend of hers asked if anyone had mistaken my head for a ball! Ouch. But that gives me an idea. A tattoo of three finger-sized holes at the top ... Still, I think I can get away with the look (without the holes that is), and there are whispers that some people even find bald heads on men attractive. Loss of hair, I imagine, is easier for men than for women. When my wife had chemo a good many years ago, she tried to embrace the Sinéad O'Connor look, but it was not so easy. There were far more strange glances to contend with. I'll enjoy the privilege of looking OK bald for a while longer, before I grow it all back.

49
Feeling the Love ... and the Likes

If you are feeling down about the number of responses that you get to your Facebook posts, simply announcing that you have had cancer or some other life-threatening disease, for example, one that requires a stem cell transplant, is a sure-fire way to up your likes. It worked like a charm for me! Seriously, when I went public on Facebook, the outpouring of well-wishes was enormous. And subsequent photos (in which I am starting to look better, I dare say) have garnered far more than the historic average of likes for me. And then there's the excessive flattery that you really want to believe. It's a good example of one of the very good roles that social media can play. There are so many people that we care about who are not directly in our lives, with whom we maintain some kind of connection via social media, hearing mostly about the good things but occasionally about the bad too. Prior to Facebook, these friends would rise to the surface of my thoughts from time to time, but most of the time images of them slumbered just below the surface of my consciousness.

If telling people that you have a life-threatening disease that requires a risky medical procedure that could kill you is difficult, appearing before them afterwards in relatively decent shape is truly wonderful. When close friends first came to the house after I returned from the hospital, I could see the sparkle in their eyes, evidence of the worry they had experienced, the love they felt, and the wonder they now had. 'He's alive; he made it!' Recently, at the encouragement of a dear colleague, my wife and I attended a work-related BBQ where people saw me for the first time since before I had gone into the hospital. Because of the haphazard way in which I had told people what was going on with me, many had only heard it second hand, and perhaps didn't even have an accurate account of it all. When I walked in, I was overwhelmed by the expressions of love and joy. So many faces looking in wonder. 'He walks!', 'Wow, he looks pretty good for what he's been through, really, don't you think.' So many handshakes and hugs, and germs! (It was my first appearance in a large group without wearing a surgical mask.)

There is something strange but touching to realize that so many people have been worried. It has taken being in front of people, being seen by them, and recognizing that I am being seen by them, to make me fully appreciate this fact. Imagining it was not really enough. It took seeing it in people's responses to me. Jean Paul Sartre makes a lot of these kinds of experiences in his discussion of 'The Look'. It's a claim with a Hegelian lineage, but he contends that we come to understand ourselves as persons, especially in moments of shame and pride but presumably not only such experiences, by experiencing others seeing us as persons. He goes so far as to claim that, 'I am for myself only as I am a pure reference to the Other' (Sartre 1992: 343).

I've spoken about my sympathies for John Donne's Meditation XVII. Experiences in which we come to understand ourselves through others give a special meaning to the claim of not being an island. After those kinds of experiences, it's hard to dismiss the idea as a piece of sentimentalism. The experiences need not necessarily be pleasant ones; but they certainly can be, and they have been for me when I've seen the wonder and joy in the eyes of my friends and colleagues.

50
Disease, Bodily Alienation, and Transhumanism

One of the things that Havi Carel says in her excellent book *Illness* is that in serious illness, one experiences a kind of alienation from one's body. Suddenly, you recognize that things are going on, going on *in* you, that you were totally unaware of, that you can't control, and that may cause you serious harm, and that may even kill you! I recall when I was first diagnosed with *essential thrombocythemia* nineteen years ago; I was in my late 30s and living in South Africa. For over a month, I'd had a bad case of the runs. The doctors were trying to figure out what was going on with my gastrointestinal tract. And in the course of doing so, they did routine blood work. The results didn't help in figuring out what was affecting my gut, but they showed that my platelet count was way out of whack, about five times higher than normal.

Suddenly, I had other problems to worry about. I was told to take it easy. They didn't want me keeling over due to a 'thrombotic event' - think heart attack or stroke. I was told to make an appointment with a haematologist as soon as possible. Something was up with my bone marrow. Most likely a *myeloproliferative neoplasm*, a group of diseases including a kind of *leukaemia*, in which one or more of the three main kinds of blood cells proliferate. The immediate thing to do was to check for *leukaemia*, which can be done by a bone marrow biopsy - my first of many groan-inducing, eye-moistening experiences of being put under the corkscrew. *Leukaemia* is ruled out if no abnormality is found on chromosome 22, called *the Philadelphia chromosome*, because it was first discovered by researchers at the Fox Chase Cancer Centre and U Penn Medical School in the City of Brotherly Love. After several nervous days of waiting, I received the negative result.

With other possibilities also ruled out, *essential thrombocythemia* was the diagnosis of exclusion. Life with a chronic disease was the new normal for me. The good news: most people diagnosed with the disease have normal longevity. The bad news is that most people diagnosed are in their 60s and 70s. Being in my late 30s, I would have decades to live with increased risk of *acute myelogenous leukaemia* or *myelofibrosis*. (The latter tailed me on two subsequent intercontinental moves, and finally caught up with me in Germany last year.) Meanwhile, the diarrhoea had not abated. At one point, the doctors had me carrying around a bucket to gather a 24-hour sample. Imagine my pleasure! I recall distinctly feeling back then that, as a still fairly young man, my body seemed to be betraying me. Suddenly, my whole system seemed to be in mutiny.

In time, the gastro problems were abated by an enzyme treatment, and I settled into the routine of taking *anagrelide*, a platelet-reducing medication that was then new in the market. Medications are approved after rigorous trial testing, but of a test population, only a fraction of the subsequent users and not over the long term. Being among the first post-trial users of the medication, I had the satisfaction and worry of knowing that I was contributing to science by helping to discover what the long-term effects were. Subsequent studies have indicated that patients taking *anagrelide* in comparison to another drug, *hydroxy urea*, are at a higher risk of developing *myelofibrosis*.

After my *myelofibrosis* was diagnosed, I had to undergo several standard physical examinations in preparation for the stem cell transplant. A thorough dental examination revealed an abscessed front tooth. Dental infections and chemotherapy-induced dead immune systems are a bad mix. So, a week before entering the hospital, my lower front tooth was pulled, and I was given a temporary fakie. When I wear it, it is hardly noticeable, when I don't I look straight outta *Breaking Bad*. In my case, there was also some concern about possible haemorrhoids, which could be aggravated by chemotherapy-induced diarrhoea. So, the docs ordered my digestive tract to be scoped. The whole thing, all 8.5 m of it.

When I went into the examination room, they asked me if I consented to having polyps removed if any were found. 'Sure, might as well find out if I have colon cancer too!' Then, unexpectedly, they asked if I wanted to be put under a general anaesthetic or to be awake to watch it all on their high-definition screen. It would be uncomfortable, they said, but not terribly painful. My curiosity got the better of me and I chose to stay awake. Just to be clear, I had been given plenty of very effective purging medication; so things were promised to be pretty empty inside.

During the exam, there was more than one moment when, feeling the probe push from the inside of my intestinal lining, it seemed like the creature from the movie *Alien* was going to pop out of my gut. Uncomfortable, to be sure. But the high-definition view made the price of admission more than worth it. It was as if I were looking out of the window of a submarine. My insides turned out to look like an alien underwater wilderness, undulating like a mass of molluscs in the waves. How weird to look at all that watery flesh and to think, that's me. But how could it be? It's me *and* it's another world! I've never been there before; I know nothing about it. Problems could arise down there, betrayals festering into carcinogenic polyps, and I'd be none the wiser for quite a while, perhaps even for too long.

My gut is as foreign to me as the bottom of the ocean. It is its own ecosystem, teaming with microbial life, all of which I am totally unaware of most of the time, and only bluntly aware of when something goes wrong. I don't direct the undulations to do my bidding. I don't intend the flesh to carry out its digestive tasks. But I am certainly more directly dependent on that region than I am on the ocean's depths. And I can't go on very well without it doing its business. If I could have my bone marrow scoped, I would probably have a similar reaction. It's not so much that illness alienates us from our bodies, as it is that in illness, we come to appreciate that we already are alienated from many parts of our bodies. And we could not live unless we were. We could not possibly direct it all, set it to work serving our purpose. Bodily alienation makes our conscious experience possible.

Alienation from my body is bound up with my limitations. If I could control it all, I would certainly sing better, play the guitar better, and have made it into the Rock 'n' Roll Hall of Fame. My talent set would be unlimited. My physical decline would be more ordered and graceful, and perhaps even seize to exist. I could stop any nascent malignancy in its tracks by sending my immune system SWAT force out to get it. And then, with unlimited time, choices would lose their poignancy. I wouldn't have to decide between being a philosopher and a rock star. I could take 40 years to get good at one thing and 40 more to get good at another. Then move on to something completely different. Comedy, perhaps.

Various parts of me could be replaced and I could carry on just fine. Better in fact, my transplant has shown that. I have heard people marvel at what an improvement their new hips are. Bit by bit, this stuff is replaceable. And I'm not lost in the shuffle of the parts. That thought suggests one way in which bodily alienation could be fully overcome. Over time, all of my parts, piece by piece, might be replaced by polymer membranes, fibre optic cables, and semiconductors. And with each new part, a monitoring and control device might be installed, giving rise to multiple feedback loops and, importantly, full awareness and control. This would be the absence of alienation. Moreover, this post-human person would seem to enjoy several advantages. Longevity without decrepitude certainly seems appealing *caeteris paribus*.

But there is one problem. I doubt that the resulting unalienated person would be me. Somewhere along the path of transition from my biological self to that post-biological, post-human person, I worry that I would disappear. The person who results from exchanging all of my body parts seems more like someone else than me. Without my body (at all), I am nothing. If this conjecture is right, what would be in it for me to bring that post-biological person into existence? I would seem to have no personal stake in it.

One intuitively plausible, but I think ultimately unsatisfying, objection is that as long as the post-human person has my memories, it's me. If we could get the technology right, I could exist that way in my physical, post-biological, existence. In response to this, recall the character Rachael in the movie *Blade Runner.* She looks just like a human, an adult woman; she feels just like a human; and she even has memories of her childhood. But she is not biologically human. She has been constructed by the Tyrell Corporation. And she has been programmed with the memories of the daughter of the corporation's owner, Eldon Tyrell. Although she has the daughter's memories, surely she is not identical to the daughter. You agree, but maybe only insofar as the daughter is still alive. (In the movie, we don't know if that's the case.) But consider that if the daughter died, is it really the case that Rachael would suddenly, in a flash, become her? That seems far-fetched. Rachael is either her all along or never. And the former seems utterly implausible. Hence, having someone's memories seems not enough to make one that person.

My focus has been on our personal fates in overcoming our bodily alienation. Two of the most influential philosophers of the nineteenth century, Hegel and Marx, saw alienation as a great social evil. In their own different ways, they developed accounts of alienation and recommendations for how it might be overcome (Hegel 1991; Marx 1978). What about the desirability of overcoming bodily alienation on a social scale over time? Imagine generations of people in the future undergoing a gradual transformation to post-humanism. Do we have reason to see the eventual transition of our species into post-human beings in full control of their artificial bodies as attractive? Not only would people overcome bodily alienation, but also perhaps achieve eternal life. I declared that, *caeteris paribus*, longevity without decrepitude is appealing. But in this case the *caeteris* definitely are not *paribus*. For reasons of personal identity, I doubt that any particular person has reason to welcome her non-biological analogue. And I can't see why we would want to celebrate the coming-into-being of a new, artificial, non-bodily alienated, and long-living post-human race. Admittedly, however, I have not argued that we should regret it either.

Disease can be bad for all sorts of reasons - it limits our abilities, it disrupts our plans, it can be costly, and it can hurt, to name just a few. We have very good reasons to want to reduce the burden of disease both within our generation - where it is especially inequitable - and for future generations. It doesn't follow that it would be good to transcend our biological existence. A utilitarian response might be that we have a reason to desire a world with less or no physical suffering. Hence, we have a reason - perhaps an obligatory one - to seek the means, through post-human transformation, to that end.

Moreover, a disease-free post-human world might have appeal beyond convinced utilitarians. Those who take rights seriously may claim that if the outcome is better and no one's rights are violated - imagine all the replacement of parts and organs over the generations is consensual - then we have reason to pursue it. To cast the net more widely still, throw in the additional constraint that the introduction of the technology at each step along the way is consistent with realizing equality of opportunity and a fair distribution of wealth. If we could manage the just introduction of an eternal, or at least very long-living, post-humanity to take our place in a more egalitarian post-human society, wouldn't that seem like a compelling goal? The reduction of suffering due to disease and ill health is doubtless good. So, one might think that every step we take in that direction consistent with justice, short of extinguishing our humanity, is surely good. If that is true, then the last step - the humanity-extinguishing one - must also be good, right?

I am not convinced that every step would be, on the whole, good. In each case, one has to weigh the gain of disease eradication against the loss. Doubts might arise regarding whether each aspect of being human can be adequately compensated for by sophisticated machine performance. Some of the things that we accomplish seem especially valuable because we, not something else, are doing it. Two examples that come to mind are the beauty of the human voice in song and the pleasures of sexual intimacy.

Moreover, it is unclear to me that by the end, the post-human beings would be capable of conscious experience. If not, there would be no overall benefit by replacing mortal suffering humans with immortal, non-suffering post-biological zombies. Debates about consciousness are notoriously divisive among philosophers; there is no consensus view about its nature and relation to physical reality. But I don't think we can just suppose that a bunch of very sophisticated machines will be conscious. I have been assuming that these machines would be persons. In fact, if we have reason to doubt that they are conscious, we have reason to doubt that they are persons. And that certainly throws into doubt the worthiness of the aim of human replacement by post-humans.

Replacement of a great many human parts will probably produce gains for human well-being in the coming years. More profound alternations could conceivably come through the use of genetic technology. As the capacity for alteration becomes more powerful, it will be important to gain more clarity than we now have about what we can replace without losing more than we gain. Discussions about that seem to be running behind technological developments presently. No less important are the moral debates about whether the long-term aim should be healthier humans or post-humans.

51
Dem Fingernails

The great American naturalist John Muir once said, 'When we try to pick out anything by itself, we find it hitched to everything else in the Universe' (1917: 158). This is a striking expression of metaphysical holism, the idea that individual things and their properties are not isolated objects, but parts of a larger interconnected whole, a complex system in which apparently isolated objects are connected to one another by their roles in the system. Whether that's true of reality in general, I'm not going to hazard an opinion. But complex systems certainly exist, and they are especially interesting to some mathematicians, philosophers, biologists, and medical scientists.

This calls to mind a song that I learned as a school child that went like this:

> The leg bone's connected to the knee bone,
> The knee bone's connected to the thigh bone,
> The thigh bone's connected to the hip bone,
> Now shake dem skeleton bones!

The idea that parts of an organism are interconnected members of a complex system is something that patients also need to keep in mind. This was driven home to me last week when I went in for one of my now biweekly check-ups.

For quite some time now - I can't really remember for how long - I've noticed that my fingernails had an odd wave in them. Every one of my ten nails has it; it runs nearly the width of the nail. At about the midpoint, the nail dips down and then back up again. And a couple of my nails have superficial cracks in them that run the better part of their length.

These nail deformities appeared at some point in the past six months since I've been out of the hospital. I haven't given them much thought, but I have found myself rubbing my fingertips over my thumbnail to catch a wave. And I improvised an armchair oncological theory that went like this. Chemotherapy kills cancer cells because it kills quickly reproducing cells. It kills hair cells for the same reason. Fingernails are fairly quickly growing. So, the fingernail deformities are probably the legacy of chemotherapy that I received in March. The fact that my toenails are not similarly affected is explained by their comparatively slow growth.

An elegant and *a priori* plausible theory that served the purpose of satisfying me and encouraging me not to think too much about my odd fingernails. But it turns out that I will not win any Nobel prizes in medicine for the theory because it is probably just flat-out wrong. The connection is more likely to be to the immune system!

Dem Fingernails

This past week I could not see my regular post-transplant doctor because he was on vacation. Instead, I saw the doctor who oversaw my transplant. And for some reason, although I never mentioned my nails to the post-transplant doctor, I felt moved to mention them to her. To my great surprise, she wasn't impressed with my oncology. She examined my nails pretty closely, showing definite interest. And finally, she declared that the deformities were consistent with graft vs. host disease!

You might recall from some of my earlier posts that this disease, in its manifold forms, is one of the main things that doctors watch for after a stem cell transplant. It amounts to the immune system (the graft) telling some organ of my body (the host) to piss off! I've compared the immune system before to a guard dog. In *The Republic*, Plato compares the best guardians of the city to good guard dogs, friendly to their own and hostile to foreign threats (1992: 375e–76b) With graft vs. host disease, it is as if the guard dogs have confused who the foreigners are. The danger is that any organ could be targeted. Obviously, it would be dangerous if it were my brain, or my heart, or my lungs. My fingernails, not so much ... I think. I suppose that this will pass without event. The dogs will go back inside in due course. But of course, my oncological credibility is already in doubt.

The doctor and I also discussed the diarrhoea that I still suffer from periodically, and she mentioned the possibility that I've developed a case of lactose intolerance, which apparently can occur after a transplant. She told me to cut back on milk and that if I still have occasional bouts of the runs, they'll need to scope me again to see if my digestive tract might also be traumatized by snarling dogs. Having gone along for that ride once, I may choose to sleep through it a second time. But with any luck, there will be no need for that and I'll have no further details to share.

Today is the six-month anniversary of my transplant. I'm pleased to report that I've been feeling good and have just travelled to a conference for the first time since the transplant. We had some excellent discussions on the ethics and politics of climate change. Assuming more and more of the duties of work feels good.

52

Traversing the Rim of the Valley of the Shadow of Death

When I checked into the hospital, I knew that I was leaving behind a loving family life, an enriching professional routine, and the company of good friends. When the door sealed me inside the germ-controlled room, my life would be very different. I felt confident that I would emerge from the bubble eventually. I was calm about my prospects. But they were far from certain. The doctors had downgraded my survival chances from 70–80 to 60–70 percent. But apart from having blood counts that caused my GP to shake her head in dismay, I was strong and healthy. Even if I was increasingly feeling the drag of anaemia. I had exercised regularly for years, in part in anticipation of the eventual need for a transplant. And I was bolstered by the thought that the risk was worth it, given the alternative prognosis of steady decline over just a few years.

I wondered how people who are sent off to war feel? Or what it's like to descend into a coal mine every day? How do people face the risks of death that their life circumstances present to them?
I didn't feel like I was descending into the Valley of the Shadow of Death, it was more like I was traversing close to the rim. The Valley was there in plain sight, and if things went wrong, I might find myself slipping into it. But I wasn't there yet.

I had gotten close to death once before. It was in Soweto when I was watching some members of a youth theatre group that my wife and I worked with. Three teenagers stormed into the dimly lit hall waving guns and brandishing knives. They wanted the valuables of the grown-ups. But they were young, amateurish, and erratic. None of which set me at ease. They lined the children and adults against a wall. Was it to fleece us or to execute some of us? As it happened, we were standing in front of a stage curtain, behind which was a door exiting the hall. We managed to slip several children behind the curtains, and they snuck out through the door. The robbers got wise to our activities and ordered us all to lie down on the floor. That felt like an execution pose. As I laid there with my arms around sobbing children on each side, I expected to hear a shot and then immediately the lights would go out. I imagined a sharp, but very brief pain, then darkness. Yet, I found myself overcome with peace. There was nothing I could do, and I was surrounded by people who needed my comfort. I remember looking at the light streaming through the high windows at an angle towards the floor. In the light beam, bits of dust sparkled like flakes of gold as they gently floated downwards. Time slowed down. But it was all over in less than ten minutes, and then we stumbled into the bright daylight, stunned that we were still alive.

Plato records Socrates's reflection on his death at his trial. He had been falsely accused and sentenced to death on the charge of corrupting the youth of Athens. Socrates contends that we have no reason to fear death, for it is either like a dreamless sleep, like nothing at all you might say, or it is an opportunity for us to enjoy the company and conversation of our friends. Fear of death is irrational because it's doubtful that after death we'd have any experiences worthy of fearing (Plato 2002: 40c–d).

Socrates could not imagine that following death, a person would survive in some kind of eternal torment as punishment for her misdeeds. Certain Christian theologians had not yet made that terrible idea seem plausible. That view was always also subject to an internal critique. Proponents of universal salvation argued that eternal torment for a sin is inconsistent with the idea of an infinitely loving, knowing, and powerful deity. The demands of justice and of mercy might often conflict, but surely if there is a perfectly just and merciful God, no one would be assigned infinite torment for an earthly crime. Socrates's alternative of either nothing at all or nothing to be feared could be rehabilitated.

Socrates's views about death were more complicated than I have let on. He certainly wasn't cavalier about his life. But he thought that living correctly was of the utmost importance, indeed more important than whether one continued to live. And that's the thrust of his response to Crito. Because he thought he had a duty to obey the authority of the Athenian laws come what may, he was willing to accept his punishment even though it meant his death. You might disagree with his claim about the solemn duty to obey Athenian laws - I certainly would - but the idea that there are things more important than merely surviving seems right.

Towards the end of his life Martin Luther King, Jr. was remarkably prescient about his death. On the night before his murder, he said, 'Like anybody, I would like to live a long life; longevity has its place. But I'm not concerned about that now. I just want to do God's will' (King 1968) Was King strengthened by the thought of an afterlife? Perhaps. But what I find noteworthy is the idea that it is the kind of life, not life at all costs, which were most important to him.

I've wondered if that idea is not only true, but also helpful in facing down death? Suppose you are taken hostage and threatened with death unless you provide information that would lead to the death of several innocent people. Who knows what you'd actually do, but if you thought the threat is credible, death might seem better than the alternative. If one has a firm grip on what is important, death may be easier to face than the alternative of losing one's integrity.

Fortunately, life rarely presents most of us with such dramatic circumstances. Terminal disease takes us away, sometimes slowly and almost certainly without fanfare. Or we confront the choice of whether to have a risky medical procedure. Or we live on with the risks that our chronic diseases pose. In comparison to Socrates and King, our lives and deaths are usually pretty mundane.

We are probably biologically hardwired to fear death, at least the immediate threat of it. Our ancestors who feared death would have been more likely to survive and reproduce. Some amount of death anxiety is probably natural. But our genetic inheritance, if there is one, would only need to trigger fear in situations of physical conflict. Having a deadly disease, I can assure you, is not quite as exhilarating as having a big carnivore bearing down on you. There is no reason to think that fight-or-flight must kick in with a bad prognosis. This is good news because it suggests the possibility of some control over fear in illness.

Socrates aimed to convince with arguments that the fear of death is irrational. Would accepting his conclusions really help with the fear? His view - or Plato's anyway - is that it can, that our emotions can listen to our reason. We are not simply at the mercy of our emotional responses, but we can cultivate a measure of rational control over them. That sort of rational therapeutic approach to fear is also a central theme in the writings of the Stoic philosopher Epictetus. If that sort of rational therapy is possible, the conclusion that there really is no reason to fear death would suggest the possibility of facing death with a measure of equanimity.

One of the things about death that is strangely disconcerting is that it's forever. When the lights go out for each of us, the universe will continue to exist for a very, very long time, and for the entirety of that time each of us will be absent. Entertaining that thought can be like placing yourself on the precipice of a very high tower. But it's not so clear why that's so. There is nothing similarly disconcerting about the thought that it all went on for a very, very long time before any of us arrived on the scene. When I read Roman history, I am not overcome with dread that I did not exist. Why is a future in which I'm absent more disconcerting than a past without me? Perhaps because some small part of that future could have been mine, but won't be. I might have lived a little bit longer, adding an infinitesimally small unit of time to a life whose duration is already puny from a cosmological point of view. But that tiny extra bit that could have been mine doesn't really seem all that significant. It's hard to avoid the thought that there is some narcissism at work when vertigo arises from the thought of an infinite future without us. If that's correct, this is another place where philosophical therapy might help with the control of our emotional responses.

The fear of death is often the fear of dying. Loss of capacity can be demoralizing. And pain really is fearful. Both of these are, however, less certain than death itself. Dying need not always include either of them. We can often reasonably hope to avoid loss of capacity and pain. And the legitimate fear of these things speaks in favour of putting patients in control of the end of their lives.

There is no trail available to us other than one of those that traverse the rim of the Valley, and one day each of us will slip. Knowing that, some try anxiously to avoid thinking about it, while others anxiously dwell on it. Rational therapy for our emotions aims for a third response. There is something to be gained from keeping in mind that the path does not go on forever; for the rarity of the opportunities afforded us is a reason to treasure them. Yet, anxiety can inhibit our capacity to do so. Not only is there often little to fear, but also fearing itself undermines the quality of the life that fear aims to protect.

53 The Examined Illness

In the record of the trial of Socrates, when he is given a chance to seek some sort of commuted sentence instead of the death penalty, he is uninterested in pleading for a lesser penalty.

Alternatives that would prohibit him from living as an itinerant philosopher in Athens are especially uninteresting because, he claims, the unexamined life is not worth living (Plato 2002: 38a). I have long despaired at the way that phrase seems to have been unreflectively appropriated by many members of my profession.

I think Socrates's famous claim is both false and disastrous for public relations, and it's not because I disvalue the examined life. Rather, I think that there are many ways to live well. I try to live mine well without disvaluing many other perfectly reasonable and admirable choices. I certainly do not believe that I have chosen the only life worth living. But I have lived with the conviction that rationally examining one's life helps it go better, even if it isn't necessary to make life worth living. And I've taken that approach with my illness. In these pages, I've tried to pursue an examined approach to my experience of illness, treatment, and recovery.

When I started writing, I didn't know whether I would survive. I approached my circumstances unable to accept the consolations of thoughts like 'it would all work out for the best', or 'it was happening for a reason'. The reason it was happening was that my bone marrow was diseased. Nothing more. Disease and serious illness often strike quite randomly. And when they do, we quickly become subject to the impersonal forces of biochemistry and pharmacology; we must trust in the training, competence, and goodwill of strangers known to patients as 'their doctors and nurses'. We rarely think about this beforehand and are usually totally unprepared for it when it happens. Suddenly, there we are, yet another patient subject to a standard treatment protocol.

Before, during, and after my 28-day hospital stay, I wrote journal entries that comprise this book. I planned them initially to be blog entries to keep family and friends informed and to keep me busy. It was to be my project in the hospital. I thought that if I had to suffer that experience, then maybe I could make something come of it. I wanted to write something that would be good. Even if I didn't survive, if in the end it was mostly just suffering and loss, it wouldn't only be that; there would be my record, which maybe would be good, I hoped. Not that it would make the whole thing worthwhile. But on balance, objectively, it would be better than without the writing.

I recognize that's a pretty impersonal way to think about it. As soon as I started writing in the hospital, I found that I depended on it. I depended on the routine. Some days, it was not easy to sit at the table and write in the midst of the fog and fatigue of chemotherapy. But that routine was part of an effort to exert a modicum of self-assertion during a time in which I was otherwise rendered nearly completely a patient. My living room/bedroom was somebody's workspace, my schedule was somebody's work routine, my immune system was being systematically crushed, and my prognosis was out of my hands.

I also depended on the writing in another unexpected way. I would usually start writing in the late afternoon and write till suppertime. I might make a revision or two after eating, and then I would upload my account of the day's activities and my condition to my blog. I would read or watch TV, knowing that around the world, at the end of the day over a glass of wine or while commuting to work on the train with a cup of coffee, people were reading. I'd lie in bed at night knowing that I was in people's thoughts, concerns, and prayers. I was not alone. Come morning, the replies would already have begun to trickle in. I was buoyed by the good wishes and the conversation. Even in that sterile and locked-down hospital room in a distant country, far from so many family and friends, I wasn't living in isolation.

It seems fair to ask what an examined illness can teach. I hesitate to say much that might be conceived as advice because I realize that it could have been much worse, indeed that it often is much worse for people with diseases similar to mine. I had it comparatively easy. The oncological psychotherapist in the transplant unit told me of a patient who had been there, mostly in isolation, for six months. I certainly had not earned an advanced certificate in suffering or staring down the grim reaper till he blinks.

True, most people do not engage in activities that stand a 40 percent chance of killing them. But, in light of the alternative, most anyone would have taken the risks that I did. I did nothing remarkable in that regard. I don't at all stand out by my choice. I also am not really responsible for the good outcome. All I did was follow my doctors' orders, more or less. I haven't honed a talent for surviving, although that would be welcome.

My illness and recovery have, however, been an occasion to think about living well, even under the threat of death. I never felt particularly angry about what befell me. And if I had, I would have hoped that I would have realized the absurdity of that, since in my case there was no person or no agency to blame. I've felt nothing but appreciation for most of my doctors and all of my nurses. I found that the experience of putting myself wholly into the trust of others for my care caused me to feel tremendous gratitude for their competence and goodwill. I also feel enormous gratitude to the stranger who was willing to donate his stem cells and thereby save my life.

And I am grateful for the fine system of payroll-tax-financed health insurance in Germany. Systems like the German one are pillars of post-war European social democracy. Their importance both for what they do, and what they say about what humanity is capable of, really cannot be overemphasized. Not only do these systems provide excellent healthcare for everyone regardless of income, but they also show that mobilization in the service of intelligent institutional design can promote the well-being of everyone.

Driven by fear, greed, glory, and the lust for power, humans have kicked up wicked whirlwinds of violence and destruction. Even as I write, parts of the world seem trapped in desperate civil wars, conditions of life described by Thomas Hobbes as, 'solitary, poor, nasty, brutish, and short' (1996: 89). Often, these end only when the war-makers suffer complete exhaustion, populations have been decimated, and survivors have been scattered as desperate refugees far from home. Who among us has not been tempted by cynicism when being confronted with the pain and despair that humans are capable of creating? But the pillars of social democracy provide evidence that intelligent design and investment can produce institutions that channel human motivation for the broad benefit of humanity. Perhaps we can do even better than social democracy. There is certainly room for improvement as inequality is growing in all social democracies. Nevertheless, its achievements should be appreciated, even celebrated, especially for indicating that humans are capable of so much more and better than war and destruction.

I have no doubt that my doctors and nurses are caring people. They are motivated to help others. But they are also interested in making a living, enjoying vacations, supporting their families, advancing their careers, and being recognized for their contribution to science and to their clinic. Social democratic institutions are especially significant because they have been able to harness human motivation for tremendous human benefit.

In preparation for the end of the US Civil War, Abraham Lincoln reminded Americans that they can live as friends and not only as enemies, and that doing so requires nothing less than activating the better angels of our nature (1861). Cynicism is a creeping disease that steals hearts already suffering pain and loss. It is also sometimes a fashionable stance of the well-educated who have known very little about such loss. The better angels are too weak, the cynic sneers. One tonic against the corrosive influence of cynicism is to keep alive in what

Lincoln called 'the mystic chords of memory' our tremendous accomplishments, including the development, advancement, and application of medical science to the benefit of humanity.

The project of living well isn't just for the healthy. Living well includes living well with disease and eventually living well facing death. I asked my wife to write an epilogue if this memoir was cut short by my death. Thankfully, it wasn't.

My illness was rare; my suffering was not. Being a patient is part of being alive. Nearly all of us go through it eventually. The virtues of patience, courage, trust, and hope serve us well. And a measure of good humour can't hurt. All of that I've learned by experience, and I hope that this record of examining my illness gives witness to what I have learned.

Epilogue: Living with Mortality

The memoir left off before the first anniversary of my transplant. In the subsequent months, I found the normalcy of the healthy life that I longed for was not as simple as I had imagined. About eighteen months after the transplant, my marriage of 29 years rapidly fell apart. My therapist, who specializes in working with blood cancer patients, told me it was not all that unusual for partnerships to break down under the stress of sickness, transplant, and recovery. Suddenly, the future seemed much less clear to me than the one I had dreamed of while sick. I had been confident in a life that was not to be. I was shaken, left unsure of what, if anything, could replace it. But I did eventually find new love and a new perspective.

As it turned out, one bout of blood cancer did not insure me against future bouts. After seven years of good health, with all of the biochemical indications positive for several years, my transplanted immune system unexpectedly and rapidly began to fail. My original immune system came creeping back, and with it the cancer. Strangely, however, not in its pre-transplant form of *myelofibrosis*, the scarring of the bone marrow that inhibits the production of blood cells, but rather in the form of advanced *myelodysplasia syndrome* (MDS), which is characterized by the production of blood cells that fail to mature, leaving blood counts, and, as I experienced it, especially haemoglobin counts, low. The anaemia left me exhausted and head-achy.

The only long-term cure for advanced MDS is the same as for *myelofibrosis*, a stem cell transplant. So, very quickly, after so many years, I was back in the transplant protocol. A search for an anonymous donor was conducted. One was found, and a couple of months later I was admitted to the same hospital as before, where once again I received a week of intensive chemotherapy to kill my sickly immune system, hopefully once and for all. After the first transplant, I came out of the hospital frail and vulnerable to germs. I was warned that the second transplant and recovery would feel harder. It did. Plenty harder. More fatigue, nausea, and dizziness; and flaming gout that consigned me to a wheelchair and then a walker for a few days.

I had expected to finish this memoir with an epilogue written at arm's length from deadly disease. Instead, I have been writing it while recovering from the second transplant. I can't offer the cool voice of reason that might come from some distance removed. Rather, cancer, chemotherapy, transplant, and recovery have always been near me as I have laboured over these sentences. At times, exhaustion has prevented me from working as I would have wanted, and a chemo-addled brain has produced confused paragraphs requiring much reworking. But the work of honing this text has been part of the struggle to re-emerge fit for the daily routine.

During both experiences of illness, treatment, and recovery, I attempted to use writing to come to terms with my circumstances. In response to deadly disease and the confusion and emotional turmoil that it produces, writing has served as a disciplined form of thinking through the challenges and as a search for a response that makes sense. I used the term 'rational therapy' in some of the previous sections to refer to this approach. I adopted the approach, not as a thesis that I was consciously trying to demonstrate, but more as a commitment to facing the problems of life, including the problems of illness. Although I was not entirely conscious of it at the time, I think much of that approach was an effort of self-preservation. I don't mean that in the sense of an attempt to survive physically, even though I certainly hoped for that, but as an effort to maintain my sense of self, not to let the disease destroy me and who I wanted to be. I think this memoir could be read as a struggle for a kind of good life even on the edge of life.

****

I owe my life to the gift of two stem cell donors. When the first one donated his cells, he was a stranger to me. He remained so for two years. Under German law, the identities of donors and recipients can be revealed to one another but only after two years and only if both parties agree. This is not the case for all European countries; in several countries, it is forbidden to disclose the identity of the parties, regardless of their will. I will never be allowed to know the identity of the donor for my second transplant because he comes from a country in which that is not legally permitted.

By chance, there was to be a meeting of European stem cell transplant specialists hosted by my university almost exactly two years after my first transplant. My doctor asked me if I would agree to meet my donor on stage. The idea was that making the meeting public might encourage representatives of some countries to reconsider their prohibition on such meetings by showing them that it can be a deeply moving experience. If more countries allowed such meetings, perhaps it would have the effect of encouraging more people to register to donate and more lives would be saved.

Despite the reality TV character of the whole thing, I didn't have to think about my response;

I immediately agreed to meet my donor on stage. Curiosity, wanting to say thank you, and helping to enlarge the pool of donors all motivated me. I attended the event with my son. We arrived early and walked together around the convention centre. I looked in anticipation, wondering if I might spot someone who seemed likely to be my donor. How I thought I might recognize him is now beyond me. The search, of course, proved futile. As the time for the event approached, we were escorted to a place in the hall where the meeting was to occur. I continued to look around to see if someone else was being escorted to a seat in the audience. I expected to see a young couple, man and woman, in their early 30s sitting nervously together somewhere. No luck. Finally, I was called to the stage. I had agreed to say a few words in German and English. I introduced myself in German and then read from my memoir. I chose the entry from the day of my transplant called 'Communion' (Chapter 13). As I read, I was nervously aware that my identity had been revealed to him, but I still did not know who among the 70 or so people in the audience he was. Finally, he was asked to take the stage as well. Frank and I embraced. He was invited to come to the podium and speak, but overcome with emotion, he declined.

Within a few months of our meeting, I visited Frank and his extended family. Later, he came to visit me for the first time. We've repeated these meetings over the years. We also text often, sharing the events of the weekend and pictures, and we talk from time to time on the phone. We have become friends, and because of our common stem cells (until my second transplant), he fondly refers to us as brothers.

What do you owe the person who has saved your life? There is a huge chasm between the ease of the act of donating stem cells and the opportunity for life that the donation offers the recipient. For the donor, the process is not especially onerous. The donation itself is easy as drawing blood. Prior to the donation, the donor must inject himself or herself with a drug twice a day for several days in order to boost the production of stem cells that will be harvested. This can induce sleepiness. For the recipient, however, the donation means everything.

Beneficence and gratitude have a place in a social field of reciprocal duties between people. In the usual case, a person renders help to another; the person helped incurs a duty of gratitude, which, when fulfilled, restores, the account between them. There is something of an economy of beneficence and gratitude. The moral equilibrium is re-established by a repayment of roughly equal measure and in the same or a convertible coin, say, a lunch in return for a drive to the doctor's office.

The economy of beneficence and gratitude holds considerable intuitive appeal in a great many cases of help offered and received. But it fits poorly in cases of a stem cell donor and a recipient.

Circumstances in which repayment of the value of the gift received will be possible only in exceptional cases. What Frank donated to me was something quite different than a lift to the doctor's office. It was not discrete; it was not even a thing in the ordinary sense. My life in its entirety, after my transplant, I owe to Frank. A coin commensurate with that gift does not exist.

Immanuel Kant discusses the gratitude children owe to their parents. Filial love, Kant holds, should 'awaken in them [the children] the determination to love their parents' (1997: 27:671). Acts of love by children expressive of their gratitude are typically appropriate throughout their lives. Now the relationship between a donor and a recipient is not one based on familial love. But their relationship shares with the relationship between child and parent the feature that one party owes its existence to the other. In both cases, goodwill expressed reliably over the course of a life is a kind of repayment for the gift of life.

Most likely, one can never fully repay the debt of gratitude to the person who has saved your life, who has given you another lease on life. Anything one does is too small in comparison to what one enjoys. The gratitude is too immense to be expressed in any individual action. This is similar to the gratitude that Kant thinks we all should have to God, as creator. According to Kant, it is the 'generality of nature' for which we should be grateful to God, not for any 'particular circumstances' (1997: 27:320). To God, according to Kant, we owe our lives. This is no individual, discrete thing or service. Rather, it is the condition of the possibility of receiving anything else.

When it is impossible to match fully the good a person has done for you, the economy of beneficence and gratitude described above breaks down. When one's life is a gift, the beneficent act is much like grace. When one has been given a life, the question of how to live in light of that arises. The expression 'living gratefully' arises naturally, I think. But here, the gratitude extends beyond the person who has given you the possibility of living. It certainly stretches the ordinary usage of the term 'gratitude' to use it without a specific intentional object, without a particular person or corporate agent in mind. But the thought that one has been given back one's life invites that way of thinking. Theologically, grace is reserved for that which is received but not earned, an object of faith or perhaps of hope. But this is the condition of my life, known to me, not merely hoped for. From here on out, life is a gift.

****

Hope, patience, and trust are all important in the lives of patients. It is not always easy to know when hope is appropriate and when it is misplaced. Hope can be an important source of inspiration; it can boost both mood and motivation. For patients, hope can help them to persevere in difficult times. I described the battle to choke down food when the mucus in my mouth and throat had dried, and nausea churned in my gut. It was the image of a stronger and healthier version of me - and the nurses' threat to put me on a nutritional drip - that provided me with the motivation to continue to eat. As I wrote at the time, hope kept me eating.

I now think it is more accurate to say my hope partially *consisted* in eating, for there is an important kind of hope that, as St. Thomas Aquinas claimed, is a movement towards the imagined good. Hoping of this kind is not inert but includes activity in pursuit of its object. Hope of this sort is much like the activity of a sculptor pursuing form by pounding it out of the rough rock of reality. Because he understood reality to be often resistant to our hopeful efforts, St. Thomas characterized hope as irascible (Aquinas 2017: II, Question 40). If the objective were easily achieved, we needn't hope. Hope, then, isn't for the faint-hearted.

I would now refer to hope of the kind just described as 'agency-hope', since it consists among other things in acting. Insofar as realizing the object of agency-hope is an achievement, this form of hoping is importantly connected to our self-esteem. Ernst Bloch posited a connection between hope and self-esteem. He argued that 'there is never anything soft about conscious-known hope'. The self-esteem that is involved in hoping is embodied in a posture.

'Walking upright is the pre-supposed, a will which refuses to be outvoted by anything that has already become; it has its preserve in this upright posture' (Bloch 1986: 147).

Aquinas and Bloch are surely right that one important kind of hope involves acting in pursuit of the hoped-for end. But we do also hope when things are beyond our influence. I may tell fellow fans how much I hope our football team will win, even though I'll only be watching the game on TV, not in any way contributing to the victory. This kind of hoping is much like wishing, except that unlike wishing, hoping is limited to what we believe to be possible. Often, patients who are subject to a demanding medical protocol have little leeway to do anything other than what their doctors order. Their agency-hope is constrained mostly to following directives. But wish-hope can be as expansive as the possibilities they imagine for themselves: sand, sunshine, and the complete absence of nausea instead of dark and rainy winter days in central Germany.

When a person takes on a hope, like any other attitude, rationality requires that it cohere with her other attitudes and actions. This suggests the idea that there are personal opportunity costs of hoping. Anyone who hopes for a team's victory cannot cheer its defeat. And if you hope to win someone's confidence, you can't sit by and do nothing to encourage it. The personal opportunity costs of agency-hope include both forgoing contradictory intentions and actions and adopting some contributory ones. Whether one should adopt an agency-hope then depends on consideration of the intentions and actions that would have to be rejected and on those that would have to be adopted in order to serve the pursuit of the hope. Since wish-hoping makes no demands of action, its personal opportunity costs are lower.

Personal opportunity costs are relevant to patients as well. In my case, there seemed to be nothing lost in working for my health by eating even when food was unappealing. There was also nothing that counted against exercising in my room even when fatigue limited my capacity to do so. But not all cases are so clear. The philosopher Adrienne M. Martin describes the fictional case of Bess, who has 'advanced and likely terminal cancer'. She signs up for an early phase clinical trial, with the information that 'there is less than 1 percent chance [she] will receive any medical benefit'. Bess reports that 'the bare possibility [of a cure] is what keeps her going, and often appeals to hope as a justification for enrolling in the trial' (Martin 2014: 14–15). Martin suggests that many people would have the strong intuition that Bess's hope is rational (2014: 16).

I think we should know more about what Bess forgoes in maintaining that hope before we agree with Martin's judgement. Bess's incredibly long-shot hope for a cure from an early-stage clinical trial may come at the expense of other valuable actions. If, for example, hoping for a cure prevents her from preparing for her imminent death, say, by making appropriate financial arrangements or by having reconciling discussions with family members, then the rationality of the hope is doubtful.

There are times in the course of an illness in which acceptance of an incurable disease can be more rational than hoping for a cure. To accept one's imminent death can open up possibilities for deeply meaningful experiences.

****

Patience and trust take on importance due to human limitations that can't be overcome. Illness is an indication of human physical finitude, and patience and trust are appropriate responses to aspects of finitude.

There are bodily processes and procedures, especially biochemical ones, in relation to which we are basically passive. Whether an abnormality indicative of MDS occurs on my chromosome 7 is not a matter of my voluntary control. Just as I can't by sheer force of will halt my heart from beating, I also can't put my mind to it and stop the formation of genetic mutations. There is no reliable evidence of causal laws running from our intentions to the biochemistry of chromosome 7. The idea that our weal and woe depend on multiple non-conscious processes is unsettling. We may not think about it often, but our conscious and intentional life is dependent on a myriad of biochemical processes that are not on the receiving end of intention formation. The heart beating is just one example. The list is long and includes the function of all our bodily organs, each playing its role without conscious direction from the mind.

Some people imagine that we have significant intentional control over vital bodily processes, perhaps even control over the development of mutations on chromosomes. This is not only not the case; upon reflection it doesn't even seem desirable. Much of what we do and accomplish depends on concentrating intently on a specific task, digging up a patch of a garden, caring for the needs of a sick child, writing a workable piece of code, or making a plausible point in a paragraph. To do these things well, we must set a number of other tasks offline. Our lives would become much more complicated, indeed beyond our capacity to manage, if we were additionally responsible for controlling the functioning of all our bodily organs.

Because we are unable to will our bodily biochemistry to behave as we would like, when it doesn't so behave, we submit to people with greater expertise regarding our bodies and with the pharmacological and technological means to manipulate the body's processes in ways that we on our own can't. As patients, we end up waiting a good deal of the time for the actions and results of others who attempt to exercise deliberate diagnostic and curative interventions. This includes waiting for test results to confirm a diagnosis, waiting for evidence of the effects of a therapy, and even waiting to see a doctor. In all these cases, we are passive *vis-à-vis* professionals in various roles of the medical industry. Our passivity is because there is a whole world of biochemical processes occurring beyond the horizon of our conscious control.

The terms 'patient' and 'patience' have the same Latin root, *pati*, which means *to suffer*. Patience is an uncomfortable virtue; the circumstances that call for it are unwelcome. Due to our limitations of agency and knowledge, we cannot get what we want exactly when we want it. The Stoic philosopher Epictetus counselled that we should direct our efforts and our caring investments only in things that we can control. This would free us from the anxiety and frustrations of directing our efforts toward matters beyond our control (Epictetus 1983: 1). According to this view, the path of happiness and freedom consists in limiting our will only to that which can be affected by our efforts.

One of the limitations that humans usually learn to live with in the course of growing up is that things beyond their full control do not happen as quickly as they would like. An omnipotent being would not have to come to terms with such waiting. For such a being, there would be no unwanted delay between willing and its outcome. For the rest of us, patience is an attitude applicable to the period of delay.

Part of being patient involves acceptance of our limitations, not railing against them. I am not claiming that patience is always called for. Some things can and should be done more quickly, and sometimes complaints help. But because we are incapable of willing into existence the outcome we want, patience will always be something we need. Without it, we can obsess about what will occur in the future, so much so that thinking about the future dominates our minds and destroys our capacity to enjoy the present. And, again because we are not omnipotent, when that future arrives, it might not be what we wanted. I have had the experience of impatiently waiting for test results only finally to receive news that was unwelcome. This seems doubly bad. It is bad enough that the results were not what I had wanted. There was nothing I could do about that. But my impatience unnecessarily made the waiting period worse than it needed to be. Knowing this to be the case helps us to motivate patience. This is central to rational therapy. Patience allows us to salvage more of the present when we can't control either what the future holds or when it will arrive.

Processes unfold in our bodies over time, and the direction that they will take is only predictable within probability ranges. Diagnosing them takes time. Responding to them can be slow. And measuring the effectiveness of the response is not immediate. Meanwhile, our lives go on. Epictetus's advice that worry has to do with things in an imagined future, not in the present, is important in this regard (1983: 5). It is a reminder to focus on the time at hand, not to let an indeterminate imagined future rob us of the present. It is, then, a corollary to his teaching to direct our efforts to what is in our control. To the extent that the future is beyond our influence, we should pay it as little regard as possible. This is not counsel to forgo planning, since planning is one way to influence the future. It is, however, advice to leave off focus on the future once there is nothing else to prepare. It would be best to remind oneself that one has done what one can, and to return one's attention to the present.

The advice of Epictetus has much to recommend when it comes to our attitudes about our own well-being. The idea that we should strive to let go of that which we can't influence is good advice against restless worry about matters that are beyond our control. It seems much less appropriate when it comes to the well-being of those in our lives whom we love. It was Epictetus, after all, who also recommended indifference towards the death of one's son (1983: 11). Such callousness is incompatible with love. This might be why the theologian Paul Tillich once claimed that the major alternative to Stoicism in western thought is Christianity, which calls for de-centring the self through acts and attitudes of love towards one's neighbours (2000: 9–17). While it would be wrong to suggest Christianity has an exclusive role in presenting this alternative to

Stoicism, it is correct to point to the problem that Stoicism has with love. When we love another person, our own well-being is vulnerable to the assaults that the beloved suffers. bell hooks puts it well. 'The practice of love offers no place of safety. We risk loss, hurt, pain. We risk being acted upon by forces beyond our control' (hooks 1999: 153). The cost of Epictetus's narrowing of concern to that which one can control is the dramatic narrowing of one's love.

David Hume counts patience among the social virtues, which are important for their 'tendency to serve the person possessed of, without any magnificent claim to public and social desert' (1998: 53). Curiously, the record of Kant's lectures suggests that he is far less impressed with patience. He praises manliness, or *animus masculus*, as 'the ability to endure evil, and likewise the hardship of life, without discontent'. Its opposite is flabbiness, or *animus effeminatus*. The gender-coded contrast of the Latin terms is noteworthy. But there is more. In an extraordinary move, he also claims that in between manliness and flabbiness is 'a female virtue', patience, which is 'the ability to get used to suffering hardships'. The difference between feminine patience and manliness seems to be that in patience 'no powers are employed to resist [hardships]' (Kant 1997: 27:646). In so attributing getting used to suffering hardships to women, Kant fully disregards the protests of his time that were led by women. To note, in surveying the food riots of the eighteenth century, the historian E. P. Thompson observes: 'In dozens of cases it is the same - the women pelting an unpopular dealer with his own potatoes, or cunningly combining fury with the calculation that they had slightly greater immunity than the men from the retaliation of the authorities' (1991: 233). Kant's failure to appreciate the agency of women is certainly noteworthy, but for the present discussion I mean to focus on his own categorical preference for resisting all forms of hardship, which, given the contrast he assumes, entails minimizing the importance of patience.

Although resistance, especially to injustice, is often admirable, Kant does not countenance that there are things in life that can only be suffered, at least for a while. If he practiced what he preached, and I suppose he did, he must have been an impossible patient. Just imagine a person of Kantian virtue in a twenty-first-century bureaucratic medical system, imperiously demanding that medical professionals provide instantaneous results for medical tests and schedule necessary procedures immediately. I imagine that this would not produce an eagerness to help.

If patience is a way of accommodating oneself to certain processes that are beyond one's capacity to influence, epistemic trust is a matter of responding to the circumstance in which expert knowledge is required to respond appropriately. This is also much needed by patients. Epistemic trust in the better capacity of one's doctors to assess and respond to one's condition is fundamental to the therapeutic process. Unless a patient is an expert in the particular branch of medicine, they can't hope to be better able to assess what should be done to treat their condition than their doctor. Both patience and trust, then, are needed due to the limitations of patient capacity. We place our trust in others when we assent to their action on our behalf or defer to their judgement regarding what we should do. If we can't do it at all, do it well, or do it in a timely manner on our own, then we have to rely on others. Just as an omnipotent being has no need for patience, neither does an omnipotent and omniscient being have a need for trust. It is because we are neither of these that there are times in which we must trust.

Trust has certain objective conditions. Obviously, we shouldn't place our trust in others when it is unreasonable to believe that they have the means and the will to achieve our end. I have had no bad experiences of medical malpractice or discrimination from medical professionals. So, in general, trust in the medical system comes easily to me. However, due to the history of medical abuse, especially against people of colour, indigenous people, women, and the poor, many patients will have a well-founded distrust of the medical system and the caregivers in it. In such cases, medical professionals have work to do to seek to mitigate the reasonable distrust so that patients have reason to trust them.

****

In the midst of coming to grips with a discouraging diagnosis or feeling very bad due to the illness or treatment, people sometimes search for a point to their suffering. The search is not directed to the kinds of answers provided by medical science, not, for example, to the role of environmental hazards or genetic predispositions in causing cancer. Appealing to these factors is similar to saying that smoking causes cancer or that the burning of fossil fuels causes storms; the cancer and the storms are made more likely by the smoking and fossil fuel use. Such causal explanations are true probabilistically. But those kinds of explanations are general. They don't answer why the particular person became ill, why environmental hazards affected her and not her neighbour, or why the genetic predisposition caused her to suffer, but not her siblings.

More importantly, explanations appealing to environmental and genetic factors tell us nothing about what sense to make of our suffering. Anyone asking about the point of their suffering is not mainly, or at all, asking for a causal explanation. The questioner is searching for an interpretation of the illness that reveals its moral importance and thereby facilitates a kind of transcendence from the misery of suffering. Perhaps the universe is trying to teach the sick person something. Or perhaps the disease is some kind of divine test. The search seems to be for the doings of a super-agent (God, the universe, etc.) that has for some reason picked out the person to suffer.

Asking about the point of the suffering appears to express a hope for a kind of transcendence of one's suffering through understanding its purpose. I find it hard not to be sympathetic to that inclination. The suffering of illness can be miserable, even debilitating. Knowing that there was a purpose for it could perhaps make it easier to bear. The philosopher and social critic, Theodor W. Adorno, once wrote that, 'Transcendence feeds on nothing but experiences we have in immanence' (2007: 398). Still, I think the question about the point of the suffering is misplaced.

The most super of all agents causing or allowing suffering would be God. If there were any other agents intervening to cause suffering, then it would have to be with the permission of an all-knowing, all-powerful being, assuming the existence of one. But when you add infinitely loving to the set of God's qualities, the thought that God would test someone with a disease seems outrageous. If you love your dog, you would never dream of subjecting it to suffering as some sort of test of its loyalty. The idea that a capricious God wants to make some people suffer, people who (on average) are surely no worse than the rest, is flat out incompatible with the three features I mentioned.

Suffering has long been thought to pose a serious theological challenge. Theologians have been involved in a centuries-long discussion of theodicy. This is the effort to explain how it could be possible for a perfect God to permit human suffering. The problem is widely considered as one of the most serious challenges to monotheism. The common assumption in this discussion is that events and outcomes in the natural world unfold according to processes that can be studied and understood by the natural sciences. When a person suffers, there is, at least in principle, an explanation of the causes that science could provide. No supernatural force directly causes suffering. It is the result of natural causes accessible to science. The question that theodicy grapples with is why a perfect God would create it in such a way that events and outcomes produce suffering? (see Hick 1990: 39–55). I'm not interested here in assessing the answers given to the question, rather I merely want to point out that even according to the theologians who have devoted a great deal of attention to the issue of human suffering, the basic assumption is that it could not be due to direct divine intervention.

Most of us take our health and happiness to be important. We invest attention and effort into living healthily with the hope of a long life. And we recognize that these matters are important for ourselves personally, but also for others, and that these are appropriate serious concerns of public policy, even of justice. So, it's not all that surprising that we should look for answers to the question of suffering in ourselves and others.

Moreover, serious illness can be debilitating either over the short term due to the rigors of the treatment or over the long term due to the morbidity it causes. Our agency and our sense of our personhood can be challenged by the mental and physical suffering that illness causes. A search for transcendence in these circumstances seems understandable even if asking about the point of the suffering is misdirected. There is, I think, another way to think about transcendence in the context of illness, and that is in our responses to our suffering.

When I was most ill, I felt in danger of losing myself to the illness, as I mentioned above, not in the sense of dying, but in the sense of becoming someone I did not want to be. One way to understand talk of 'battling' or 'beating cancer' is not in terms of being cured, but in terms of self-preservation. In this alternative understanding, a person may battle cancer and win even while succumbing to it physically. Battling in this sense involves jealously clinging to oneself, one's remaining agency, and struggling to preserve one's personhood. Audre Lorde's comments in this regard inspire. 'It was important for me, after my mastectomy, to develop and encourage my own internal sense of power. I needed to rally my energies in such a way as to imagine myself as a fighter resisting rather than as a passive victim of suffering' (Lorde 1980: 73).

Understanding the point of suffering is not the only form that transcendence can take. Drawing upon one's own sense of power, even while the doctors and the medicine take the curative lead, is also a form of transcendence, a form of resistance to the immanence of suffering.

****

Loss of oneself can come in many ways. Disorientation and demoralization can result from considering one's physical finitude and the ultimate end that such temporal limitation spells to all of one's pursuits. Can it all still matter if eventually I will die in any case? A possibly deadly disease brings one into confrontation with the fact of one's eventual death in a way that is unavoidable. Even if mortality was something one had managed mostly to deny up to that point, it's very difficult to do so when the whole point of the rigorous medical procedures that one has agreed to is aimed at extending one's life.

The philosopher Cheshire Calhoun's discussion of demoralization, although not directed towards one's mortality, seems relevant here. She describes the way that loss of confidence in one's power of instrumental reasoning can be demoralizing:

> For most of us, most of the time, the insecurity of life against disastrous misfortune is a fact to which we do not consciously attend and that we do not affectively register. But when the background frame of confidence in the hospitableness of the world to ongoing human agency is disrupted, one may lose

> the sense that deliberation has a point. In sum, we lead our lives under an idea of our future - of who we will be and what life circumstance we will find ourselves in. Taking a motivating interest in our own future depends on our being able to sustain an idea of our future under which future-oriented desiring, hoping, aiming, and planning make sense.
>
> (Calhoun 2018: 66)

Mortality puts the final brakes on our projects of instrumental reasoning. Knowing that participation in relationships and in one's projects must eventually come to an end might encourage doubts about whether it makes sense to continue to pursue them. This would be a depressing conclusion.

One might think that a religious belief in the afterlife offers a neat response to that depressing conclusion. In Christianity, the writings of the Apostle Paul are appealed to as support for the hope that there is, or will be, a resurrection in the form of a spiritual body (1 Corinthians 15 1987). This would be a form of continued individual identity, embodied in some way but not physically so, and not in space and time. Like many theologians, the philosopher of religion John Hick understands some form of afterlife as required by any plausible theological answer to the problems of theodicy mentioned above. The problem that a redeeming afterlife responds to is that over the millennia, countless millions of people have lived and died in conditions of extreme misery. Hick interprets the great world religions as presenting a view of the universe as soteriological, which is to say that the universe contains some form of redemption available to everyone, even those innumerable many who lived and died mostly in wretched conditions of serfdom, slavery, warfare, and grinding poverty. Hick writes:

> However pervaded by suffering the lives of hundreds of millions have been and are, and however unrealised their human potential, those lives as seen by the post-axial faiths [the world religions] nevertheless all have their place in a soteriologically structured universe. Their gospels declare that the project of human existence is not meaningless and in vain.
>
> (1989: 61)

The attraction of an afterlife according to this view is the opportunity it poses for a kind of salvation for what otherwise looks like the hopeless fate to which so many people in human history have been consigned, a fate that is hard to reconcile with the idea of a perfect God.

Importantly, however, Hick insists that because a resurrection as understood by Christians necessarily requires divine intervention, death is something Christians rightly fear.

> The religious difference between the Platonic belief in the immortality of the soul, and the

> Judaic-Christian belief in the resurrection of the body is that the latter postulates a special divine act of recreation. This produces a sense of utter dependence upon God in the hour of death ... Hence, in the Jewish and Christian conception, death is something real and fearful.
>
> (Hick 1973: 101)

Hick's view is consistent with the reported final words of Jesus on the cross, crying out that he's been forsaken (see Mark 15:34 1987; Matthew 27:46 1987). If a religious commitment to an afterlife is not strong enough stuff to overcome fear of death, then it would seem unlikely to offer sufficient help with demoralization in the face of mortality.

An alternative kind of immortality, less miraculous than personal resurrection, is to think that little bits of energy or consciousness might disassemble from the current configuration that constitutes us and then continue to exist in some other form. Perhaps the bits of consciousness become parts of several new lumps in a cosmic stew. But just as my body doesn't continue to exist after I die, when plants and animals consume and metabolize its parts, so it seems that my identity would also no longer exist if the bits of my consciousness dispersed and became constituents of other conscious beings. Belief in this kind of afterlife then would also seem unable to counter demoralization caused by an awareness of mortality.

Perhaps we make too much of our mortality. The philosopher Bernard Williams thought so. He argued that living forever would be unbearably tedious (Williams 1973: 82–100). He claims that this would be so because we would run out of projects that would be sufficiently important to us. Williams calls these 'ground projects'. He believes that there is a limited number of any such projects a person can have in a life, and that commitment to them serves to unify a person's identity over the course of that life. Once we have completed all the projects we have, which must happen, he claims, over an infinite time horizon, life would become insufferably boring.

Williams seems to have a very peculiar view of what counts as ground projects, certainly one that I don't share. For him, maintaining friendly and loving relations doesn't seem to count. But fostering, participating in, and caring for loving relationships and friendships are among our most important projects. It is an occasion for deep sadness when death brings these projects to an end, and it would be wonderful if they did not have to end. Contrary to Williams, I can't fathom how immortal life could be tedious if I could maintain my most cherished relationships forever.

A different possibility for responding to demoralization draws on the arguments of the philosopher Derek Parfit. He argues that our attitudes about our mortality have their source in an irrational preference for the future over the past. The more rational attitude is that of a character that Parfit refers to as Timeless (Parfit 1986: 173). Timeless is indifferent to whether the good things in life are in the past or in the future and therefore is far less bothered by the finitude of life looking forward. 'As our life passes, we should have less and less to look forward to, but more and more to look backward to.' Parfit believes that if we were not biased towards the future, the circumstance of a limited future would not be a source of unhappiness because memories of the past grow as expectations for the future diminish.

Parfit's view also strikes me as implausible. It is meant to have a normative punch - we *should* reorient our thinking backwards and worry less about the future. But the view that we really ought not to be so future-oriented depends on whether an alternative is possible for us. *Ought* implies *can*. Philosophers as diverse as Ernst Bloch, John Dewey, and Martin Heidegger, among others, argue that looking forward is a fundamental feature of our experience (1986: 4; 1917: 13; 1962: 279). We are committed to the future; we pursue plans that orient our lives. And recently, a number of social scientists have argued that our basic orientation towards the future is part of our evolutionary heritage, not something we can simply jettison. We are biologically disposed to prospection (Segelman et al. 2016). These considerations suggest that, even if Timeless were happier than we are, his is not a point of view that we can adopt, and therefore not a way for us to live with mortality.

So, what then is a good response to the threat of demoralization about our mortality? In the course of the experiences recorded in this book, I was relatively hopeful about my survival prospects. Not at every moment, of course, but for the most part. I had confidence in the competence of my medical team and my chances of surviving. When I was first diagnosed with the return of cancer and the need for a second transplant, the possibility of failure loomed in my mind in the way that it did not the first time. When writing about it at the time, I referred to my thinking as being in the grips of 'a pessimistic fallacy'. The fallacy is in thinking my likelihood of surviving a second transplant must be far lower than surviving the first one. If the survival rate of a single transplant is, say, 70 percent, then the chances of surviving two are 35 percent. Nonetheless, I had to bring myself not to lose sight of the fact that the likelihood of surviving the second one was also 70 percent, no lower than the first time.

I mention my response to the pessimistic fallacy as an example that shows that to some extent, our attitudes about our illness are within our rational control. Not necessarily immediately, perhaps not fully and certainly not without work, but nonetheless, we possess some capacity to adjust our responses. That suggests that a kind of rational therapy is available to us. When we are demoralized or afraid, it can help to consider whether our emotions are appropriate in light of what we know about the circumstances. Epictetus, as I have mentioned, had confidence in this kind of rational therapy. If we aim to be happy and free of worry, we should focus our attention on outcomes that are within our control, and not on those that are not.

The best response to demoralization in the face of mortality is, I think, to understand that the finitude of our lives gives each of us reason to value our lives and our project more than we do already. Why is this? Each of our own lives is rare in the sense that they are singular and finite. This sort of argument has a general application: rarity gives us a reason to value even more the things that we already have reason to value. The fact that an engaging piece of art is singular and very much unlike any other increases its aesthetic value and provides us with a reason to take special care with respect to it. As with art, so with our own lives. Our mortality gives each of us all the more reason for valuing our lives and the activities that comprise them. A similar argument can be made about fragility. We have reason to take extra care regarding fragile things that we have reason to value.

I live with and care for an old dog. Rex has been my companion for fourteen years. I adopted him as a puppy, and he has accompanied me through an international move, divorce and new love, and two experiences with cancer and stem cell transplants. Given his age, I am very much aware of his mortality. Caring for him has been an important project in my life. The fact that it will soon come to an end is not in any way a reason to stop caring. On the contrary, I value the time that I have with him even more, precisely because I am aware that there is not much more of it left.

In one of the only books written by a philosopher on illness, Havi Carel comes to a similar conclusion. 'Appreciating our finitude enables us to live each moment with full appreciation of its distinctiveness and the weight of responsibility implied by this view' (Carel 2008: 117). That the time ahead of us is limited is an additional reason to value it. Carel's claim that each moment is distinct should not, however, be misunderstood. Appreciating the rare value of our lives doesn't entail viewing every experience as valuable. That would be overreaching. Recall the analogy to art. Valuing a rare work of art doesn't entail the judgement that it is flawless in every regard.
I raise this not as a logical curiosity, nor out of a special interest in the fallacy of division. The argument for the value added by rarity applies only to things we already have reason to value. It is very important to understand this in regard to end-of-life decisions. There may be moments in a valuable life, even extended periods, that we have no reason to value. If when looking ahead, one is confronted with the prospect of relentless and severe pain or progressive loss of capacity and fatal illness, one might have sufficient reason to want a valuable life to end.

The rational therapy suggested by Epictetus is premised on the assumption that our responses to our mortality are to some extent under our control. Even though we all have experiences of irrational responses and desires, recognizing them as such and focusing on what we have reason to value can be helpful in managing pessimism and demoralization.

There is a question of how much of our response to mortality is in principle modifiable by a kind of Stoic-inspired rational therapy. Existentialist thinkers often emphasize (rightly, I think) the prospective nature of our experience. On the final horizon of all prospection is death. Hence, we are unavoidably confronted with our mortality once we begin thinking about our lives as a whole. Death completes our lives by bringing it to an end. As we think about how we ought to live, we are then faced with our mortality. But we live, the existentialists argue, without final authoritative guidance from pattern or prescription. Existentialists reject the idea that there is a species-specific form of human flourishing or the good life, as Aristotle and others have claimed (2009: I.7).

In contrast, the life aims or plans available to us are contingent, usually based on custom and choice. They are not required by any basic truth about human excellence. So, in confronting our mortality, we face up to the contingency of the life plans we pursue, and we confront the thought that our lives involve an arbitrary pursuit of aims that can't be grounded beyond contingent facts about ourselves. I imagine the resulting anxiety a bit like the distress of Wile E. Coyote, who, in pursuit of the Road

Runner, finds himself hanging in the air beyond the edge of the cliff. He realizes that here is nothing to ground him. This is the human condition, according to existentialists. Anxiety is not a mood that might pass or a pathology that one could be cured of. Tillich refers to this as the anxiety of meaninglessness (2000: 47)

According to this view, anxiety is not a bug that is fixable; it's a feature. No amount of rational therapy is going to relieve us of our anxiety. Efforts to do that would seem deeply delusional. That our death lies before us as something certain but unchosen, something we are 'thrown' into, is for Martin Heidegger what gives rise to our anxiety about death. Death is what human existence ends in and so anxiety about death is anxiety about our 'potentiality for being' (Heidegger 1962: 295).

Although according to Heidegger, anxiety is not a mood, the use of the term 'anxiety' would not track our usage unless it had an affective state, something similar to fear but without a specific object. Anxiety is not just the cognitive understanding that our deepest commitments, what Williams might call our 'ground projects', are ultimately contingent. However, the argumentative move from recognizing such contingency to affirming the necessary existence of anxiety seems to be precisely the problem spot for this account.

My intellectual recognition that the well-being of my son, one of my most important concerns, is contingent first on my having fathered him and second on living in a culture in which parental responsibility is deeply ingrained, doesn't produce anxiety in me. Perhaps the existentialist's point is that anxiety results from recognizing such contingency in *all* of my deepest commitments. But why and how? When I was preparing for my transplant, I was worried about my death in regards to my son. But my worry took the form of a specific fear about his well-being, not anxiety about my potentiality for being.

Where does this leave us? It leaves me unconvinced about the existentialists' claims about anxiety. If a reader of Heidegger objects that they don't experience life in the way he describes, it seems that his only responses would be to doubt either their understanding of their experience or their sincerity. The first seems presumptuous and the second insulting. Other philosophers have imagined that we can live reasonably happily without being grounded in a basic truth of human flourishing. John Stuart Mill, for example, celebrated experiments in living precisely in the absence of knowledge about what the ultimate good is (1879: Chapter 2).

A return of cancer after one has survived it can be deeply demoralizing. With the first diagnosis of cancer, one's awareness of one's own mortality takes on prominence in one's experience. If the therapy is successful in containing the threat, over time one's awareness of one's mortality is just one feature of a busy life, not dominant but present. But after a visit to the doctor and the discussion of bad test results, suddenly mortality is back in the forefront of the mind. There is the realization that even if one survives a second experience of cancer with a decent prognosis, there is no cosmic ledger sheet that ensures that there will not be a third one. And in any case, whether death comes by cancer or by some other means, life will come to an end, and with it all the aims and projects that one pursued with love, enthusiasm, and commitment. This is living with mortality.

I have thought of my mortality as shadowing me ever since my late 30s, when I was first diagnosed with *essential thrombocythemia.* Back then, the doctor said he had good news and bad news. The bad news was the disease itself, a kind of *myelodysplastic syndrome.* We know these colloquially as blood cancers. The good news was that most people diagnosed with that particular disease have a normal life expectancy. Oh, but there was one more piece of bad news: most of these people are in their 70s, so I should not be surprised if the disease transitioned to *myelogenous leukaemia* or *myelofibrosis* one day, at which point my chronic condition would become acute. Mortality has seemed to me a bit like Zarathustra's shadow in Nietzsche's *Thus Spoke Zarathustra.* The shadow says to Zarathustra at one point: 'But after you, oh Zarathustra, I've flown and followed longest, and even when I concealed myself from you, I was still your shadow; wherever you sat, I sat too' (Nietzsche 2006: 221).

If recognition of our mortality is a permanent feature of our lives, always accompanying us like Zarathustra's shadow, we can nonetheless develop various responses to it. As Lorde says: 'There must be some way to integrate death into living, neither ignoring it nor giving in to it' (1980: 13). Death also hangs over my relationship with Rex, but, as I have insisted, that is a reason for me to value our remaining time together all the more, not to stop caring for him.

Navigating a life neither obsessed with nor in denial of one's mortality is a tricky business. An awareness of our mortality can, and, I have argued, should give us reason to value what is good in our lives even more. And knowing that we only have one life to live can help frame the importance of some decisions; there are goals that will never be pursued if the opportunity to do so is put off too many times. Not facing up to the limits on our time then leads to a kind of mistake in appreciating value and opportunity. But giving undue attention to our finitude can also lead to a fear that robs us of appreciation of the value and opportunities that exist in our lives.

****

Zarathustra's example of living with his shadow may provide us with a model for living with mortality, but his own life is no model for our own. As Epictetus recommended, Zarathustra lives detached, without deep connections to others. Connections of friendship and love enrich our lives, but they are also the source of tremendous suffering and grief. There is no escaping the sadness of serious illness and death. In her beautiful poem, *In Blackwater Woods*, Mary Oliver writes,

> To live in this world
> you must be able
> to do three things:
> to love what is mortal;
> to hold it
> against your bones knowing
> your own life depends on it;
> and, when the time comes to let it go,
> to let it go.
>
> (1983: 82)

We don't escape the grief of mortality. Such grief is not demoralization and not depression; it is the tribute we pay to what we value, what has been meaningful in our lives. When one is seriously ill and the risk of death is very high, the idea that our relationships will end is an occasion of sadness. Sadness not because a patient must learn to live without those who have enriched her life. No, it's that her loved ones may have to let go of her. The sadness of loved ones reaches the patient by the chords of sympathy that Hume described. It would be perverse and cold to argue that the ill person ought not be sad because she will not experience the loss of a relationship in death. Nor should the loved ones feign a lack of sadness, for the grief is nothing more than an expression of love. And there is grief in serious illness even if one avoids death because in such illness we confront our own fragility and the frailty of our most valuable relationships. This is the pain of living, of loving. I have survived humbled and with a far greater sense of my fragility.

In interpreting my own experience, much has not been very clear until I have articulated it, and even then not fully clear. Finding the right words is part of settling on an understanding. Language brings things into focus that are inchoate and in flux until expressed, but there is also a need to fit the words to the experience. I'm not free to just make up how I felt and responded. That would be the route of self-deception and delusion. But the touchstones of my felt experiences and response are also interpretations. And so, the effort is steeped in ambiguity. My effort at understanding my experience seems necessarily to have shaped it.

Writing this epilogue has been a struggle with words to express broader insight. I have hoped that both the memoir and the epilogue are about more than *my* experience. But the effort to achieve broader insight is especially difficult. I'm not confident that I have succeeded. That will be for readers to decide. The text may be mostly a record of, and insight into, my own disposition. Nothing more. It has been an attempt to make sense of my illness, treatment, and recovery and to orient myself in the onslaught of fear and confusion that comes with a very serious illness. Writing helped me to try to be the person I wanted to be. My self-preservation, not just my mortality, has been at stake. I can't escape that first-person possessive adjective when describing the effort. Surely, much of what I say here is peculiar to my personality, not all that useful to others. So, just as I have tried to examine my illness, examining my text is necessary to determine if insight about more than my perspective can be found. Still, writing the text helped me; I hope that reading it helps you.

As I emerge now with a third lease on life, I hope that my resolve to learn from and to improve the world is at least as strong as it was before my two transplants, and that my sense of wonder and my capacity for love remain intact. It didn't take cancer to teach me the importance of these, but I would not want it to cause me to forget.

References

1 Corinthians 15 (1987), King James Bible, Red Letter ed., Nashville, TN: Thomas Nelson.

Adorno, Theodor W. (2007), *Negative Dialectics*, New York: Continuum International.

Aquinas, Thomas (2017), *Summa Theologica* (trans. Fathers of the English Dominican Province), New Advent, https://www.newadvent.org/summa/. Accessed 15 July 2025.

Aristotle (2009), *Nicomachean Ethics* (trans. W. D. Ross and L. Brown), Oxford: Oxford University Press.

Aurelius, Marcus (2017), *Meditations* (trans. G. Long), Mineola, NY: Dover Publications.

Bloch, Ernst (1986), *The Principle of Hope,* vol. 1 (trans. N. Plaice, S. Plaice and P. Knight), Cambridge, MA: MIT Press.

Bloch, Ernst (1995), *The Principle of Hope* (trans. N. Plaice, S. Plaice and P. Knight), Cambridge, MA: MIT Press.

Bodhi, Bodhi. (trans.) (2000), *The Connected Discourses of the Buddha: A New Translation of the Samyutta Nikāya*, vol. 2, Somerville, MA: Wisdom Publications.

Calhoun, Cheshire (2018), *Doing Valuable Time: The Present, the Future, and Meaningful Living*, Oxford: Oxford University Press.

Carel, Havi (2008), *Illness: The Cry of the Flesh*, Abingdon and New York: Routledge.

Dewey, John (1917), 'The need for recovery in philosophy,' in J. Dewey (ed.), *Creative Intelligence: Essays in the Pragmatic Attitude*, New York: Henry Holt, pp. 3–69.

Donne, John (1999), *Devotions Upon Emergent Occasions and Death's Duel* (ed. A. Clements). Oxford: Oxford University Press.

Ecclesiastes 9:7–12 (1987), King James Bible, Red Letter ed., Nashville, TN: Thomas Nelson.

Epictetus (1916), 'Discourses', in *Discourses and Enchiridion* (ed. G. Long, trans. E. Carter), London: George Bell & Sons, pp. 3–375.

Epictetus (1983), *The Enchiridion* (trans. E. Carter), Amherst, NY: Prometheus Books.

European Medicines Agency (n.d.), 'Jakavi', https://www.ema.europa.eu/en/medicines/human/EPAR/jakavi. Accessed 11 June 2025.

Gawande, Atul (2014), *Being Mortal: Death and What Matters in the End*, London: Profile Books.

Hegel, Georg Wilhelm Friedrich (1991), *Elements of the Philosophy of Right* (trans. A. W. Wood), Cambridge: Cambridge University Press.

Heidegger, Martin (1962), *Being and Time*, Oxford and Cambridge, MA: Blackwell.

Hesiod (1914), *The Homeric Hymns and Homerica* (trans. H. G. Evelyn-White), Cambridge, MA and London: Harvard University Press and William Heinemann Ltd.

References

Hick, John (1973), *The Philosophy of Religion*, Upper Saddle River, NJ: Prentice Hall.

Hick, John (1989), *An Interpretation of Religion: Human Responses to the Transcendent*, Basingstoke: Palgrave Macmillan.

Hobbes, Thomas (1996), *Leviathan* (ed. R. Tuck), Cambridge: Cambridge University Press.

hooks, bell (1999), *All About Love: New Visions*, New York: William Morrow and Company.

Horace (2004), *The Complete Odes and Epodes* (trans. D. West), Oxford: Oxford University Press.

Hume, David (1998), *An Enquiry Concerning the Principles of Morals* (ed. T. L. Beauchamp), Oxford: Oxford University Press.

Kant, Immanuel (1996), *Metaphysics of Morals* (ed. and trans. M. Gregor), Cambridge: Cambridge University Press.

Kant, Immanuel (1997), *Lectures on Ethics* (ed. P. Heath and J. B. Schneewind, trans. P. Heath), Cambridge: Cambridge University Press.

King, Martin Luther Jr. (1968), *I've Been to the Mountaintop,* Memphis, TN: Mason Temple, 3 April [Speech], Stanford University, The Martin Luther King, Jr. Research and Education Institute. https://kinginstitute.stanford.edu/ive-been-mountaintop. Accessed 4 December 2025.

Lincoln, Abraham (1861), *First Inaugural Address*, The American Presidency Project, 4 March, https://www.presidency.ucsb.edu/documents/inaugural-address-0. Accessed 11 June 2025.

Lorde, Audre 1980, *The Cancer Journals*, San Francisco, CA: Spinsters/Aunt Lute.

Mark 15:34 (1987), King James Bible, Red Letter ed., Nashville, TN: Thomas Nelson.

Martin, Adrienne M. (2014), *How We Hope: A Moral Psychology*, Princeton, NJ: Princeton University Press.

Marx, Karl (1978), *Economic and Philosophic Manuscripts of 1844* (trans. M. Milligan), Amherst, NY: Prometheus Books.

Matthew 6:28–34 (1987), King James Bible, Red Letter ed., Nashville, TN: Thomas Nelson.

Matthew 27:46 (1987), King James Bible, Red Letter ed., Nashville, TN: Thomas Nelson.

Mill, John Stuart (1879), *On Liberty and the Subjection of Women,* New York: Henry Holt and Co.

Mill, John Stuart (2004), *Utilitarianism* (ed. R. Crisp), Oxford: Oxford University Press.

Muir, John (1917), *My First Summer in the Sierra*, Boston, MA and New York: Houghton Mifflin Company.

Nietzsche, Friedrich (1996), *Human, All Too Human: A Book for Free Spirits* (trans. R. J. Hollingdale), Cambridge: Cambridge University Press.

Nietzsche, Friedrich (2006), *Thus Spoke Zarathustra,* Cambridge: Cambridge University Press.

Nunes, Kelly et al. (2020), 'How Ancestry Influences the Chances of Finding Unrelated Donors: An Investigation in Admixed Brazilians', *Frontiers in Immunology*, 11:584950, https://doi.org/10.3389/fimmu.2020.584950.

Oliver, Mary (1983), 'In Blackwater Woods', in *American Primitive*, Boston, MA: Back Bay Books, pp. 82–83.

Parfit, Derek (1986), *Reasons and Persons,* Oxford: Oxford University Press.

Parker, Theodore (1853), 'Of justice and the conscience', in *Ten Sermons of Religion,* Boston, MA and New York:

Crosby, Nichols, and Company and Charles S. Francis and Company, pp. 66–101.

Plato (1967), *Gorgias, in Plato in Twelve Volumes*, vol. 3 (trans. W. R. M. Lamb), Cambridge, MA and London: Harvard University Press and William Heinemann Ltd, pp. 447–527 (original work written *c.*380 BCE).

Plato (1992), *Republic* (trans. G. M. A. Grube), Indianapolis, IN: Hackett Publishing (original work written *c.*375 BCE).

Plato (2002), 'Apology', in *Five Dialogues* (trans. G. M. A. Grube), Indianapolis, IN: Hackett Publishing, pp. 21–44 (original work written *c.*399 BCE).

Proverbs 16:18 (1987), King James Bible, Red Letter ed., Nashville, TN: Thomas Nelson.

Ryan, Paul (2017), interviewed by H. Hewitt, *The Hugh Hewitt Show*, Salem Radio Network, 10 March.

Sartre, Jean-Paul (1992), *Being and Nothingness: An Essay in Phenomenological Ontology* (trans. H. E. Barnes), New York: Washington Square Press.

Schmidt, Alexader H. (2024), 'Unrelated hematopoietic stem cell donor registries: present reality and future prospects', *Current Opinion in Hematology*, 31:6, pp. 251–260, https://doi.org/10.1097/MOH.0000000000000835.

Segelman, Martin E. P., Railton, Peter, Baumeister, Roy F. and Sripada, Chandra (2016), *Homo Prospectus*, Oxford: Oxford University Press.

Springsteen, Bruce (1984), 'No surrender', *Born in the U.S.A.*, CD, New York: Columbia.

The Commonwealth Fund (2015), *U.S. Health Care from a Global Perspective: Spending, Use of Services, Prices and*

Health in 13 Countries, Issues in International Health Policy, New York: The Commonwealth Fund.

Thompson, Edward P. (1991), *Customs in Common*, London: Penguin Books.

Tillich, Paul (2000), *The Courage to Be*, New Haven, CT: Yale University Press.

T. S. Eliot (1943), 'Little Gidding', in *Four Quartets,* New York: Harcourt, Brace and Company, pp. 21–39.

UIC Today (2016), 'Medicare to cover stem cell transplantation for sickle cell disease', 7 April 2016, https://today.uic.edu/medicare-to-cover-stem-cell-transplantation-for-sickle-cell-disease/. Accessed 4 December 2025.

Wikipedia (2025), 'Fludarabine', https://en.wikipedia.org/wiki/Fludarabine. Accessed 11 June 2025.

Williams, Bernard (1973), 'The Makropulos case: Reflections on the tedium of immortality', in *Problems of the Self*, Cambridge: Cambridge University Press.

World Health Organization (2014), 'World Health Statistics 2014', 15 May, https://www.who.int/news-room/detail/15-05-2014-world-health-statistics-2014?.com. Accessed 11 June 2025.